# WHY COUNT SHEEP WHEN YOU CAN SLEEP?

The Read-in-Bed Guide
for Getting Your Zzzzzs

Tracy Ecclesine Ivie

Attention corporations, associations and other organizations. Contact the publisher to use our books as fundraisers, premiums or gifts.

Rose Street Press
Box 244
Annandale, NJ 08801
908-730-0355 I www.rosestreetpress.com

Cover design by Genevieve LaVo Cosdon

Library of Congress Control Number: 2010903311

Ivie, Tracy Ecclesine
Why count sheep when you can sleep? The read-in-bed guide for getting your zzzzzs / Tracy Ecclesine Ivie

ISBN 978-0-9843711-0-5


10 9 8 7 6 5 4 3 2 1

ii

# Why Count Sheep When You Can Sleep?

To Bill, Doug, Kitty and Eve

To Margy and Joe, wherever you are—
parents, free spirits and writers extraordinaire

This book is also dedicated to the millions of
people who face a common enemy every night. May
you find peace in these pages…

# Contents

# Why Count Sheep When You Can Sleep?

## Introduction

Welcome to *my* world—another night married to the snorer from hell.

A freight train is bearing down on me from a foot away. Chug. Chug. Chug. Gasp. Honk…Gasp.

I nudge his arm. No response.

I shake his shoulder.

"Huhhhhhhh? Huhhhhhhh? Wha-a-a-?"

"You're snoring, Bill."

"Huhhhhhh?"

"You're snoring."

"Snor…ing?"

"Yes, snoring."

"Oh." (He turns over.)

Silence.

# Introduction

But now I'm in overdrive—worries on parade.

"I wish my daughter would stop smoking and going to tanning booths. What if I have to raise her children?" (*Note: She doesn't have any yet.*)

"Where'd I put the key to the safe deposit box?"

"I'm overwhelmed with work. What if I miss a deadline?"

"What if I got really sick?

"Will I *ever* finish this book?"

And so on...

I try to quiet my mind by breathing v-e-r-y slowly, counting each breath as the air goes in and out: one...two...three... Somewhere around 3:15, I start drifting off.

Honk...honk...chug....gasp. There it is again, louder than ever.

I'm awake, I'm asleep, I'm awake, asleep...

Ad infinitum.

It only took us about 30 years to discover my husband has sleep apnea. He literally stops breathing about 28 times an hour every night. So now he wears a "CPAP" (pronounced see-pap) mask with a long nozzle that looks like something out of an old

# Why Count Sheep When You Can Sleep?

"Sea Hunt" rerun on TV. The CPAP feeds air into his lungs, making a soft whooshing sound that rarely wakes me up.

Unfortunately, however, I still wake up in the middle of the night sometimes. Old habits die hard.

## Turning off my mind

But now I have a solution—*this* book.

During all those years of lying awake, I frantically searched for ways to lull myself back to sleep. I read lots of books and articles about insomnia, but most of them were much too clinical.

Besides, I didn't want to read about insomnia BEFORE I went to bed or AFTER I woke up. I needed something right then and there, while I was desperately alone at night, grasping for anything that would put me back to sleep (as long as it wasn't sleeping pills, since I didn't want to go that route).

I wanted an "in-bed" guide filled with sleep tips I could use when my mind was racing. Since I'm a writer, I vowed to write the definitive book myself—especially when I found out that more than 40 million people in the United States alone also can't get a good night's sleep.

That's a lot of people searching for solutions. And I wanted to help…

# Introduction

## Alone in the dark

I started with variations on the old "counting sheep" routine, going backwards and forwards, and slower and faster. I did the same thing with breathing exercises, creative visualizations and even "in-bed" calisthenics (which I think I invented), boring, repetitive exercises designed to numb my mind back to sleep.

I made a list of things that worked and before I knew it, I had quite a collection, my own personal menu of sleep tips I could turn to whenever I needed. No more wracking my brain trying to remember what worked.

But I wanted more tips for this book, so I contacted relatives, friends, business associates and even total strangers on the Internet, asking for solutions. And even though my original purpose was to write a book for getting back to sleep in the middle of the night—without ever leaving the bed—I expanded my focus to include the beginning of the night as well as "out-of-bed" sleep remedies, since a lot of people sent great ideas for these categories.

## Read it and sleep

The best thing about "Why Count Sheep When You Can Sleep?" is that it's a collection of *real* tips from *real* people that *really* work. It's short on theory, long on practicality and the *only* insomnia book designed to be read in bed—at the point of insomnia—when you need it the most.

# Why Count Sheep When You Can Sleep?

Because no matter why you're awake (and this book is no substitute for medical advice), everyone who can't get to sleep at night is at the same place—alone in the dark, frantically searching for relief.

**The critical 20 minutes**

Experts say you should get out of bed after 20 minutes of lying awake, and "Why Count Sheep When You Can Sleep" was written for that critical time period. Think of this book as your 20-minute insomnia crutch because everything you need is right here in black and white.

And if you still can't get to sleep, check out the ideas from people who've found relief by getting out of bed and distracting themselves with other activities.

**How to use "Why Count Sheep..."**

The next time you find yourself a prisoner in your bed, anxiously watching the clock, reach for your book light, e-book reader such as a Kindle or iPod (this book is available on them too), snuggle under the covers and skim through the pages until something catches your eye. You only need one thing that works, and there's more than enough for everyone here.

The information in this book is presented in what may seem like an illogical order, but it's not. For example, the "pre-bed" (bedtime) sleep tips are at the end, not the beginning. The "in-bed" sleep tips are first because they make this book different from every other sleep book on the market. They're the heart of the book—tips to read while you're in bed, not before or after.

Plenty of other books give "pre-bed" sleep tips, which medical professionals call "sleep hygiene." Because they're so important, I'm including them. There's nothing terribly original here, particularly if you've read other sleep books, but if any of these "pre-bed" sleep tips help, then I've done my job.

Here's how "Why Count Sheep When You Can Sleep?" is arranged:

## Read-in-bed sleep tips

This section is broken down into several parts, which you can dip in and out of at will:

The first two chapters are about my two favorite sleep solutions—slow breathing and EFT (Emotional Freedom Techniques), since about 80 percent of the time that's all I need. Then comes a quick chapter on self-hypnosis and the "Relaxation Response" before we're on to the meat of the book: tips from "around the world" and then from me.

## Journal

Next up is a journal section, so you can empty your mind on paper, which is a very effective way to wind down. Many sleep experts highly recommend this, so I've given you plenty of space to record your thoughts.

# Why Count Sheep When You Can Sleep?

## 'The Boring Book'

Last in the "read-in-bed" offerings is a very special section, "The Boring Book," so you don't have to jump out of bed to find one. This little mini-book gives new meaning to the phrase, "It's a real sleeper."

"The Boring Book," as you've probably surmised, is a very tedious read. It's filled with half-formed thoughts and illusions, run-on sentences and jumbled dialogue that just doesn't hang together. Unless you have a multiple personality disorder, nothing in "The Boring Book" will make the slightest bit of sense.

## Out-of-bed remedies

These are the tips for getting back to sleep once you've left the bed to start rambling around your house. Plenty of people contributed great ideas for this section.

## Pre-bed rituals

OK, now we're finally at the beginning, a roster of widely accepted (along with some rather unconventional) pre-bed rituals that have helped many people start the evening in a more relaxed state of mind. Follow these suggestions and you may never need the rest of this book.

So with my very best wishes, I invite you to make "Why Count Sheep When You Can Sleep?" your bedside companion—your best friend when nothing else will do.

Read it and sleep.

**Medical disclaimer**

This book is not a substitute for medical advice. "Why Count Sheep When You Can Sleep?" cures nothing and is strictly a coping mechanism. Think of it as your nightly band-aid when nothing else works, a collection of ideas that have helped many people get through the night.

But that doesn't mean you should ignore any underlying medical problems. Numerous conditions can cause insomnia, including depression, heart disease, fibromyalgia and arthritis. And some sleep disorders, such as sleep apnea, are quite serious. If you snore a lot, seek professional help, which may mean visiting a sleep clinic, where you can be monitored by specialists trained to detect abnormalities.

I also recommend seeing a chiropractor, who can clear up blockages that may be contributing to a lack of sleep. The spinal column houses the spinal cord—the heart of the central nervous system—which controls every activity of the body. When the vertebrae are out of alignment, they decrease the effectiveness of the nervous system and can cause aches and pains or stress. Chiropractors can free up these blocked neural pathways so your entire body functions better, which can do wonders for your sleep.

# Why Count Sheep When You Can Sleep?

Lastly, although sleeping pills may be warranted in some short-term situations, even the manufacturers warn about overuse and side effects. Sleeping pills are, therefore, not in this book.

However, I'm including some herbal remedies recommended by various people which are generally considered safe. I'm passing along their comments for information purposes only and do not endorse any of these products, so please **use them at your own risk**. If you're taking other medications, check with your medical provider.

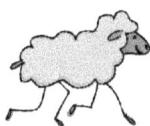

# Part I:

*Read-in-Bed Sleep Tips…and More*

# Why Count Sheep When You Can Sleep?

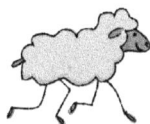

# B-R-E-A-T-H-E

# Why Count Sheep When You Can Sleep?

"Slow down, you move too fast..."

*The 59th Street Bridge Song (Feelin' Groovy)*

Why did I devote a whole chapter to breathing techniques—an entire chapter to something that takes only a few minutes?

Simply because it works so well for me. Of all the techniques in this book, slow breathing and EFT (emotional freedom techniques) are the two I turn to first, and 80 percent of the time, that's all I need.

Sometimes I even combine the two, doing a few quick rounds of EFT first to jumpstart my concentration.

Breathing jolts me back to the present moment when my mind is racing all over the planet. Sometimes it takes me almost 100 breaths before I can focus on one complete breath from start to finish because my mind is so busy churning over the events of the day or worrying about tomorrow.

What a reward to *finally* have control...

## Slow mo

Think of each breath, if you will, as an exercise in slow motion, with a beginning, a middle and an end. Take about five to eight seconds for each breath and when you finally zero in on one without interruption, congratulate yourself, whether it took you 20 breaths or 200 to get there. Keep cheering yourself on whenever you completely focus on one breath. It's an accomplishment, and you deserve to feel good about yourself. And before you know it, you'll be asleep.

**To your health**

Deep breathing promotes blood flow and digestion. It also massages our organs, including the stomach, liver and heart.

Here's a short meditation called "Breath" by Dudley Evenson, reprinted with permission from one of Daily Om's most popular online courses, "A Year of Guided Meditations." These medi-tations last about a minute and include flute playing and a short nature video (www.dailyom.com and click on "courses" or visit www.soundings.com, 800.93PEACE).

Read this slowly and deliberately, listening to the sound of each word in your mind.

BREATH

I take a deep breath, inhaling fully, holding for a moment and then exhaling slowly and completely. I feel the energy my breath brings to every cell and molecule of my being.

Inhale. Hold. Exhale. Exchanging energy. Bringing in fresh, new, life-giving energy. Letting go of what is old and used. My breath is bringing in the life force. I let go of what is unneeded. In and out.

With each breath, I am restoring and revitalizing myself. I am completely refreshed with each breath I take. I am healthy. I am alive.

## Yoga breathing

Your breath is a bridge between your body and your mind so if you can control your breath, you can control your mind. It's that simple.

Pranayama, a type of yoga breathing, controls prana, the life force. Beginning Pranayama, which I do, is a two-part belly breath. More advanced yoga students use a three-part breath that involves the entire respiratory system. I recommend you only attempt the advanced breathing under the guidance of a yoga master.

Two-part breath:

Slowly inhale through your nose (mouth closed) and keep your chest still as you expand the air into your abdomen. Let your stomach rise like a basketball. Now hold your breath for a few seconds.

Then contract your abdomen and slowly push the air all the way up your chest and out your mouth, making a blowing sound as you release the air.

# Breathing

Work your senses so the breathing becomes a slow, steady rhythm and you're watching, feeling and hearing each breath as it's taken in and released.

- Imagine there's a long tunnel between your mouth and your stomach. Now, visualize the air going into your nasal cavity, down your throat and into your abdomen. Hold your breath for a second or two in your belly and then watch the air return all the way back up and out your mouth.

- Hear the sound of your breath as it passes through your nose and quietly swirls down to your stomach. Then listen to the whooshing sound as the air is released from your mouth.

- In the meantime, place a hand on your stomach as it rises and feel yourself lightly pushing the air up and out your body.

As I breathe in and out, I usually count the breaths, aiming for about 350, if I can stay awake that long.

## Variations

Other sections of this book list breathing variations, but I wanted to mention some of them here because they're so effective.

# Why Count Sheep When You Can Sleep?

*Smiling*

It's virtually impossible to focus on your worries when you're smiling, which immediately puts you in a better frame of mind.

*Contracting your muscles*

As you breathe in, tense your entire body. Hold for a second or two and then release your muscles when you exhale. Try to do this at least 350 times.

*Progressive relaxation*

You can also tense your body in stages, for example, starting with the top of the head on your first breath, the forehead on the next and then the eyebrow, etc. Take your time... I sometimes break down the breath into miniscule sections of my body, such as the space above my upper lip, and then my top lip, bottom lip, etc., or my right earlobe, my collarbone, etc. This is what I call the slow drag-out.

Another variation is to tense parts of your body together, such as your entire head on the first breath, then your neck, chest and shoulders on the second followed by your arms and hands on the next, then your stomach, buttocks and hips and finally, your legs and feet.

*Mantra/phrases*

Each time you breathe, repeat a phrase in your mind, such as "good air in" as you inhale and "bad air out" as you exhale. Or repeat a word in your mind or a series of words. The important thing is the repetition.

"Om mani padme hum" is a traditional Buddhist mantra known for its healing properties. The mantra helps normalize breathing and calms the mind. Also look into the Buteyko breathing method, based on this mantra, which was developed for asthma and anxiety, but which supposedly helps with sleep apnea as well. www.buteyko.com

One of my recent favorites is very simple, but I'm amazed how well it works. On the in breath, I focus on the word "right" and on the out breath I think of "now," so as I'm rhythmically breathing in and out, my mind is repeating, "right now, right now, right now…"

*Visualization*

As you breathe, picture something relaxing to focus on, such as a beach with the waves crashing on shore or the view from the top of a snow-covered trail or the Grand Canyon — anything beautiful that takes you outside of yourself.

*Counting*

Count your breath with each new inhalation, so the first breath is one, the second is two, etc. Visualize each number in your mind while you're counting.

# Why Count Sheep When You Can Sleep?

There are many variations on counting. For example, count to five on the inhale, hold for four and then exhale to eight counts. You can use any numbers that feel comfortable to you.

Remember the goal is to be in the present moment, not the past or the future. With a little bit of practice, you can do it!

## Your Notes

Techniques that work for you (from the previous list—or new ones you create):

Other comments:

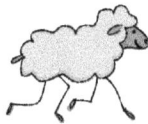

# Emotional Freedom Techniques (EFT)

# Why Count Sheep When You Can Sleep?

I love EFT and use it on many things. It's my favorite way to get back to sleep besides slow breathing. And since EFT only takes a few minutes, I often do it first to jumpstart my breathing exercises.

The Emotional Freedom Techniques were founded by Gary Craig and involve tapping on acupuncture points with your fingers to connect to your mind/body's natural healing power. EFT has been used on many physical or emotional issues and is based on the belief that "the cause of all negative emotions is a disruption in the body's energy system."

On his Web site, www.emofree.com, Craig offers a free download of the EFT manual as well as numerous other training materials.

Before getting into the process, here's a note from Jessica Ortner, who along with her brother, Nick, has created a line of educational products centered on the Emotional Freedom Techniques:

> I have a great and easy-to-learn insomnia antidote. I created a documentary film about a technique called EFT, Emotional Freedom Technique. Most people know EFT as "tapping" or "acupuncture without the needles." You literally use your fingers to tap on nine acupressure points that help you relax. In this film we follow a mother who had recently been diagnosed with breast cancer. She said the insomnia that started after the diagnosis was worse than the chemo treatment. She had

EFT (Emotional Freedom Techniques)

tried medication with no success. After filming her using EFT, her insomnia is gone and she no longer needs the medication.

Note: Besides tapping, EFT involves self-dialogue. Here are the basics:

Start by asking yourself how much of a problem you're having with insomnia (on a scale of one to 10).

Then it's time to start tapping. As you tap on each area of your body, say to yourself (aloud or in your mind): "Even though I'm having trouble sleeping, I deeply and completely love and accept myself." Repeat this phrase while you tap each area about seven times.

(Another variation of the wording is the "choices" method, developed by Dr. Patricia Carrington, which focuses on positive affirmations. Using this method, you'd say something like this while tapping: "I choose to go to sleep right now. My eyes are heavy and I feel very relaxed.")

**Tapping**

Take the index and middle finger of either hand and tap about seven times on each of the points below in sequence. As Craig says, tap solidly but not hard enough to hurt or bruise yourself. Repeat each sequence three times.

# Why Count Sheep When You Can Sleep?

It doesn't matter which side of the body you tap on. I like to alternate hands, starting with my right, and continuing a total of six complete sequences (three on each side). I usually start with my right hand, tap on each of the points below, and then do a complete round with my left hand, then right, left, etc., ending with my left hand.

Where to tap:
1. The "karate chop" point — the side of your hand between your pinky and wrist. (For example, If you're using your right hand, tap the side of your left hand, and vice versa.)

2. The eyebrow point: the inner corner of your eyebrow near the bridge of the nose. (For 2-7, I tap on the same side as my hand, and at number 8, I cross over to the other side.)

3. The eye socket bone on the outside corner of your eye. (Avoid hitting your eye!)

4. Under the center of your eye at the top of the cheekbone.

5. Halfway between the bottom of your nose and your upper lip.

6. Halfway between the bottom of your lower lip and your chin.

7. About an inch below the "U" in the center of your collarbone – at the top of the first rib.

8. Under your arm, about four inches below the armpit.

9. On the top of your head.

Now ask yourself again how much of a problem you're having with insomnia (on a scale of one to 10). I guarantee it'll be a lot less. In fact, sometimes I can feel my level drop almost three points as soon as I start tapping.

Note: According to the EFT manual, EFT should not be used on people with severe psychological disorders. Craig's Web site also states that although EFT has produced remarkable clinical results, it is considered experimental and people must take complete responsibility for using it. He offers his techniques as an ordained minister and a personal performance coach and suggests that people consult qualified health practitioners regarding their use of EFT.

## Your Notes

Techniques that work for you (from the previous list—or new ones you create):

Other comments:

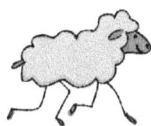

# 'The Relaxation Reponse' and Self-Hypnosis

# Why Count Sheep When You Can Sleep?

Numerous people mentioned self-hypnosis and the "Relaxation Response" in connection with insomnia.

Since this book is primarily a collection of short tips for getting to sleep, I'm only going to describe these two concepts briefly here. There are numerous books, tapes and programs on the market for further study.

Many of the tips in the following chapters are variations of the Relaxation Response and self-hypnosis.

## 'The Relaxation Response'

In 1975, Herbert Benson, M.D., published the ground-breaking book, "The Relaxation Response," about a meditative technique to help relieve anxiety. According to the book, the Relaxation Response is an altered state of consciousness that quiets the nervous system, resulting in a lower heart rate, slower breathing and decreased blood pressure, among other things.

After doing many studies on the Relaxation Response, Dr. Benson recommended that people do the technique for 10 to 20 minutes at a time, once or twice daily, for maximum relaxation. The Relaxation Response was intended to be done in a sitting position so people would stay awake. However, the book notes, if a person is lying down, he or she will most likely fall asleep.

# 'Relaxation Response' and Self-Hypnosis

In a nutshell, the technique involves being in a quiet environment, finding an object to focus on (or repeating a mantra) and ignoring distractions that pop up.

If this sounds like meditation and self-hypnosis, that's because they produce changes in the body that are similar to the Relaxation Response.

## Self-Hypnosis

Self-hypnosis is a trance-like, heightened state of awareness that allows you to control parts of your brain that are normally inaccessible by your conscious mind. You can use self-hypnosis to help reach any goal, including quieting your mind when you're trying to get to sleep.

According to the experts, self-hypnosis is similar to meditation but it includes positive "post-hypnotic suggestions" while in the trance-like state.

Here are three techniques for hypnotizing yourself:

1. Stairs:
   - Close your eyes and picture yourself at the top of 10 steps, with a door at the bottom. Each time you take a breath, feel yourself getting more relaxed as you step down toward the door.
   - Listen for the beat of your heart and quietly say the word "relax" with each succeeding breath.

- At the bottom of the steps, open the door and go to a place of deep relaxation—real or imagined—which could be a beach, meadow, waterfall or any other peaceful setting.
- Use as many senses as possible to explore your surroundings. Feel the waves pounding the shore, hear the sounds of the birds, smell the air, pick up a seashell, etc.
- Relax and enjoy the peaceful energy.
- Now imagine yourself sound asleep, without a care in the world.

2. Breathing:
   - (No steps or a door this time, just breathing.) Each time you breathe in, focus on letting go of the tension in your body, slowly working down from your head to your toes. Feel yourself getting lighter with each breath until you are floating on air.
   - Tell yourself, "I am peacefully falling asleep and feel very calm and relaxed."

3. Water vessel:
   - Slowly breathe in and out, tensing and releasing different parts of your body until you feel totally relaxed. Once you feel limp all over, imagine filling up your body with cool water, starting at your toes until you are a vessel of soothing liquid energy.
   - Picture yourself completely at peace as you drift off to sleep.

## Your Notes

Techniques that work for you (from the previous list—or new ones you create):

Other comments:

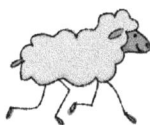

# Sleep Tips—From Around the World

# Why Count Sheep When You Can Sleep?

When my mind is racing and I'm having trouble falling back to sleep, I try to picture a beautiful lake... I focus on the surface of the water and imagine that all my thoughts are drops hitting the water. At first, it's like a hard rain, and the surface gets really rough. Then, I watch as the rain slows down and the surface becomes very still.

April Biddle

Wear a sleep mask and custom-fitted earplugs, made from a cast of the inside of your ear. These earplugs usually cost around $60 and one brand that makes them is Bernafon.

David Berman

I keep a pad by the bedside and I write down everything I'm thinking about. This helps me feel reassured that I don't have to remember it all. Once it's captured someplace else, my mind feels at ease because I know I can come back to it on paper in the morning.

If that doesn't help, I find that focusing on a singular thing does. So I will very often hold an image in my mind that has small details, such as a flower. I picture it close up and in as much detail as I can. This gives my mind something to focus on and the other distractions can fall away.

# Sleep Tips—From Around the World

Another focusing technique I use with great success is to lie in bed with my eyes closed and silently recite all the United States presidents in order from one to 44. This accomplishes the same thing—keeps my mind focused and my thoughts channeled in ONE direction, instead of jumping all over the place. It's the same premise, I suppose, as counting sheep, only sheep are so UNchallenging that my mind wanders. The focus thought has to be challenging enough that I won't mentally wander off.

Monica Ricci

The best remedy for me is to imagine two big stage curtains falling and closing, like at the end of a very long play and there are no more curtain calls. Corny, but it really works for me.

Another solution is to imagine perfect whiteness. Nothing above, nothing below, just warm comforting whiteness. It relaxes my mind and clears my thoughts. It is like wiping the screen clean and starting over. Not quite meditating, which requires more effort. This is more like putting everything on pause and hitting the "clear" button.

Natalie McCullough

Instead of counting sheep, I say the rosary and other prayers I learned as a child.

Vince Cardarelli

# Why Count Sheep When You Can Sleep?

1. Say to yourself: relax my feet, relax my ankles, etc., working all the way up to "relax my busy, busy brain." I learned this in yoga in the 1970s and used to fall asleep right there in class during shavasana (relaxation). I was a teenager, and it changed my life. I realized we have a lot more control over our bodies than we think.

2. Progesterone cream. I am on bio-identical hormone replacement therapy and I have hormone creams made up separately, estrogen and progesterone, instead of combined in one. Progesterone is the "relaxation hormone," so when I wake up in the middle of the night I just rub some extra progesterone on and it helps me get back to sleep. A weaker progesterone cream is available over the counter and also works. I used Kokoro brand before I got my prescription.

Lauren Traub

⁓

As a past sufferer of insomnia, in lieu of medicine and binge drinking, I opted to focus on the Fibonacci sequence: 0, 1, 1, 2, 3, 5, 8, 13, 21, 34*

I found that if I focus on one thing that requires my concentration—something I can do with my eyes closed—it often works. It's not 100 percent effective, but it's been about 85 percent effective for me in the past.

Bonnie Vandewater

# Sleep Tips—From Around the World

*(TEI note: Named after 13th century Italian mathematician, Leonardo Fibonacci, the Fibonacci sequence is a series of numbers in which each number is the sum of the previous two, e.g., 1+1=2; 2+1=3; 3+2=5; 5+3=8; 8+5=13; 13+8=21, etc.)*

The best thing I've found (and it's a recent find) is Bach's Sleep Remedy, a holistic spray. It helps quiet a mind that is racing due to stress. I took it on a trip and it helped so much! I slept like a baby.

Terry Traveland

I write myself to sleep at night. I call the technique sleep-writing, and I've been doing it for many years. Some of the stories I've sleepwritten were recently published in a book titled "Bedtime Stories: The short, long and tall tales of a sleepwriter."

Here's the technique: I pick up my notebook and start writing the first words that pop into my head and keep writing for three pages—no editing, no looking back. By the time I've gotten to the end of the third page, my de-stressed mind has unwound and relaxed, I can hear my own voice, my pulse has slowed and I slip into a deep and restorative sleep.

Barbara Worton

# Why Count Sheep When You Can Sleep?

For me, the iPod has been a gift straight from heaven! I keep it next to my bed. When I wake up and can't get back to sleep, I pop in the ear bud and listen to one of my relaxation, guided meditation favorites. And there are so many recorded meditations, relax-to-sleep kind of things online that I can always get new ones, try out different voices, etc. And 100 percent of the time, when I do this, I fall back to sleep! It's great.

Kara L. C. Jones

❧

Close your eyes and slowly visualize the word "S-L-E-E-P" one letter at a time as if you're skywriting in big, white puffy letters. Repeat as many times as necessary, each time slowing down the pace of the letters.

Jim Donovan

❧

You can think about gift buying, your hectic work schedule, a host of other errands you can't do and how worn out you're going to be.

Or, take a deep breath. Let it out slowly—if necessary, several times. Now, think of a peaceful time. In your mind, see yourself relaxed, still and free of stress.

Feel yourself becoming lighter, eyelids heavy. Drift off into a restful sleep. Usually, this works on the first try. If it fails, I do it again.

Marcella Glenn

I used AdrenaCalm, a skin cream sold through chiropractors. It stops the cortisol response that keeps the adrenal glands chugging away and therefore wakes you up. It works wonders for people who wake up out of a dead sleep around two in the morning. But my skin was very sensitive to it and I broke out in a rash.

Randy Peyser

Try listening to relaxing music or doing some guided imagery relaxation exercises. If possible, you might also try to address the source of the anxiety. For example, if you find that you're worried about forgetting to do something important the next day, get up and write it down. The simple act of ensuring you will remember in the morning can help you relax.

Make sure you're comfortable.

It's difficult to sleep when you're uncomfortable. If you wake up in pain or discomfort, treat the symptoms. This applies to treating physical symptoms as well as environmental ones. If you find that your room is too hot or cold, too bright or noisy,

# Why Count Sheep When You Can Sleep?

make changes so that your sleeping environment is more comfortable. When the discomfort is addressed, it will be much easier to fall asleep.

Dr. Mike Steinberg

⌒〜〜⌒

I use a couple of acupressure points with my clients—especially women in menopause —and it works very well.

K 6 is directly below the inside of the anklebone in a slight indentation and B 62 is in the first indentation directly below the outer anklebone. Squeezing these two acupressure points on each foot with your thumbs and first fingers while breathing deeply works so well that I can't even do it without falling asleep. Most of those who have tried it are pleased with the results.

Kathi Casey

⌒〜〜⌒

When insomnia raises its ugly head, I just lie there and listen to my cat Miro purr. I get my breathing in sync with his purring and before long I am back to sleep.

Pablo Solomon

# Sleep Tips—From Around the World

The two methods that work for me are:

1. Repeating in my mind the following phrase:

   "Why am I here? To sleep. So...sleep."

   Sounds so silly and simple, right? All I can tell you is that it works for me every time I seem to be having a "sleep issue."

   The challenge is keeping the mind focused on the phrase, because otherwise the mind will wander, and wander far, keeping you awake.

2. I hang a pair of small "in the ear" headphones on my ears (small enough to sleep on) and listen to what is called "ambient" music. There are Internet channels that play 100 percent ambient music 24/7, and radio programs like "Hearts of Space" that can point you toward the right sort of artists. This music often has a "drone" aspect to it, and certainly never anything surprising, shocking or emotional. It is often rhythmless (or anyway, without drums). This type of music puts me to sleep real fast. *(TEI note: Try http://somafm.com/listen and go to "Drone Zone.")*

Classical music, which was largely developed with religious sponsorship, is not a good choice, as it is full of fearful sounds, "'breakthrough" swells and triumphal charac-teristics. Even baroque music "says" too much. It's very pretentious and uplifting—not what you need when you are trying to go to

# Why Count Sheep When You Can Sleep?

sleep. Nearly all music contains "stress" and "emotion" of one nature or another, except SOME ambient music.

A lot of ambient music is not really ambient at all: It is full of sounds evocative of danger, the unknown or even loss and depression. AOL Radio's ambient channel (incongruously located in the dance-electronic category of their Web site) is one of the "not-ambient-at-all" examples. I have created a Pandora channel I call "Ambient (Classic/Electronica)" that works well most of the time. I stream it into my head using my iPhone so that I don't have to be tethered to a computer all night.

Scott Shuster

Without question, self-hypnosis and self-hypnosis CDs are ideal solutions for insomniacs. Many people find it difficult to sleep because of chronic stress and anxiety, hormone changes, depression and overstimulation of the brain with too much information and radiation (technology overdosing).

Learning how to focus on one's own breathing, just at the belly, relaxing deeper on every out breath, can be very soothing and bring attention away from the active mind. For those who aren't motivated to do it themselves or find it uncomfortable to draw their attention inward, self-hypnosis CDs can be played or uploaded onto MP3s.

Dr. Sunny Massad

# Sleep Tips—From Around the World

I read until I fall asleep. If I wake up later, I read again until I fall asleep again. Another tactic: I try to force my eyes to stay open. Eventually, they close.

MaryAnn Miller

My husband is an aural kind of guy, very into music. When he can't sleep, he plays a delta sleep CD on his CD player.

I am a visual woman so I grab my flax and lavender eye pillow and cover my eyes. At the same time, I do a deep breathing yoga/meditation exercise.

Jill Nussinow

A drop or two of lavender essential oil rubbed into my neck and/or pillow is very relaxing.

Amy Logan

I have my Walkman set to the BBC, and whenever I can't sleep, I just put in an ear bud and listen. It puts me right back to sleep.

Bob Seeley

# Why Count Sheep When You Can Sleep?

When I can't get back to sleep, I read. Also, a hot water bottle always makes me feel good. I put it between my knees or down at my feet. I also like to spray lavender all over my pillow top. It calms me down and puts me to sleep.

Lis King

I usually listen to a relaxation audio recording or do some yoga. When there's something heavy on my mind (I recommend this to my clients too), I journal in a "stream of consciousness" kind of style—it usually helps me get the thoughts out of my head and then I can go back to sleep.

In the long run, I try to eat well and exercise every day. I find that if I have abnormal meals or sit around all day and just watch TV, I have a hard time getting a full night's sleep.

Doreen Amatelli

I watch Jay Leno on DVR. Works for me.

Charles Wasilewski

I read something or get up and take the dog for a walk.

Tom Stillman

# Sleep Tips—From Around the World

I keep some magazines by the bed and when I can't sleep, I read. As long as they have nothing to do with my work, I fall right back to sleep.

Tom Davis

I try to picture a white board with nothing on it, and keep that image in my mind. Also, I take melatonin or/and calcium before going to bed. And all the obvious: pray, get up and read, write, drink water, try not to eat too close to sleeping, whatever.

On extreme nights, I'll go take a bath or check e-mail until I'm exhausted.

Amy Ecclesine

I just slather on lavender face cream by L'Occutaine on my face and body.

Anonymous

When I can't sleep, I reach for the remote control on my TV and turn it on with the sound off in the "closed caption" mode. This means I'm forced to read from the screen. I like to sleep on my side so it's really hard to stay awake when I'm concentrating so hard on reading the words sideways. I also set a timer, which

# Why Count Sheep When You Can Sleep?

turns the TV off in about an hour.

Debbie Rittelman

I'm an Eagle Scout and have taken wilderness survival courses. I sleep better when I'm outdoors, so if I'm having trouble sleeping indoors I imagine that I'm outside in the woods all alone. It's very relaxing.

Another thing that works for me is to imagine that I'm in front of a black wall and am walking toward a white light. In some weird way, that kind of relaxes me. The trick is focus on one thing—and only one thing.

John Connors

I think about the place that is the most peaceful for me and I try to experience it fully—what does it feel like, look like, smell and taste like. You've really got to work all your senses.

Ed Duffy

I have developed a flower essence blend for helping all aspects of tiredness and anything related to tiredness, and many people have told me that it helps them get to sleep, particularly in the middle of the night. My Web page lists all of the ingredients in this blend, www.nmessences.com/everyday/tiredness_mixture.html.

Flower essences are totally different than essential oils. Essential oils are produced (usually) by distilling volatile oils from plant materials whereas "flower essences" are purely an "energetic remedy" that have no biochemical action on the body. They work on the body's energy.

Peter Archer
Aromatherapist and flower essence practitioner

My insomnia tips:

Relax. The only reason we need sleep is to realign our energy. Let it be OK that you're not getting your "eight hours" of sleep. When you resist the fact that you can't sleep or have woken up in the middle of the night, it causes more tension. Even simply allowing yourself to relax will help you align your energy.

One of my favorite tricks is to intend that no matter how much sleep I get, I'll feel great in the morning. This allows me to relax. As a mother of an infant, I put this theory to the test and it works!

If I wake up in the middle of the night or can't sleep when I turn the light out, I use that time to focus on my goals. I envision how I will feel when I manifest the goal. I create more details about how I want the goal to transpire. This

# Why Count Sheep When You Can Sleep?

usually puts me to sleep within five to 10 minutes and I feel emotionally well.

Jeanna Gabellini

## Your Notes

Techniques that work for you (from the previous list—or new ones you create):

Other comments:

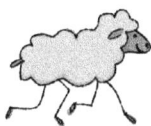

# Sleep Tips—
# From Me

# Why Count Sheep When You Can Sleep?

OK, you're awake. Now what?

Here are some of my favorite techniques for getting back to sleep in the middle of the night, but you could try them any time you can't sleep. I started the book with just these tips and then added more from people all over the world, which created a tremendous diversity of ideas.

So here they are—with love.

**Get comfortable.** Check and fix your pillow, mattress, room temperature, pajamas (too much, too little), etc. Take as much time as you need to wiggle around and adjust everything, because when your mind is agitated, you need your physical surroundings to be calm and restful. If you aren't comfortable, every little thing is just another reason to be distracted from falling back to sleep.

**Assume the cocoon position.** Think of a butterfly being formed, or a baby in its womb. Feel a warm glow encircling your body, creating a layer of insulation between you and the outside world.

You can probably do this from any position, but I usually lie on my right side. Then I tuck the covers against my neck and the small of my back as "mini-pillows" and so I'm not distracted by the flow of air. (My dog does the same thing when she sleeps, resting her body against a pillow, the side of a couch or even a shoe.)

# Sleep Tips—From Me

If you're on your side, move your chin a little closer to your chest. There's something about looking down that tends to create an even better cocoon.

**Find your "personal sleep zone."** This is really important. Make it your goal to create that spacey, semi-conscious feeling you get just before falling asleep. Think of it as your private signal that sleep is near. For me, the zone is a certain ring in my ear that symbolizes I'm about to drift off. I know exactly how it sounds and feels.

As soon as I'm comfortable in bed, I start listening for that high-pitched tone. If it's not there, I try to imagine it in my mind. You can do this with any of the exercises in this book. The sleep zone is always there waiting for you—you just have to find it.

Still awake? Move on to:

**Affirmations.** If you're having a hard time turning off your mind, repeat some of these phrases over and over, slowing down each time while imagining yourself drifting off into a dewy fog…

"My head is very heavy."
 "I'm going to sleep now."
 "I'm very tired."
 "I'm so tired."
 "Everything is going to be OK."
 "I'm a good person," etc.

Why Count Sheep When You Can Sleep?

# COUNTDOWNS

**Count sheep (and the whole rest of the menagerie)**—nothing new here, except why focus on just sheep – and why not give them something interesting to do, like jumping over a fence? (Make it fun for those damn sheep!) So if you've never imagined pink elephants, now is a good time to watch them bounding over a fence. Or for that matter, cats, dogs, monkeys or giraffes.

Remember that old song, "The Bear Jumped over the Mountain"? Well, start visualizing bears flying over Mt. Fuji or Mt. Kilimanjaro or maybe the Atlantic Ocean...the sillier the better, because it takes energy to imagine these odd things—energy you won't have to spend worrying about your life.

Now vary the tempo, counting v-e-r-y s-l-o-w-l-y, and then if you get bored, speed it up for a while and then go back. Don't forget that if you get to 350 and you're still awake, try 500 and then 1,000. And then start counting backwards.

**Count numbers.** Did you ever see those old black and white TV newsreels, where the numbers zip down from 10 to 1 in a big circle? Try picturing that image with a new number from 1 to 350 each time, v-e-r-y s-l-o-w-l-y.

Or imagine big, bold numbers and no circle. Now count to 350, excruciatingly s-l-o-w-l-y. Or try puffy cloud numbers or pink

59

polka dot numerals. It's up to you, whatever you feel like watching that night.

**Count people.** (Variety is the spice of sleep.) Every time you say a new number, imagine another face. Try to let the faces dissolve into one another. Now vary the tempo so you're counting v-e-r-y s-l-o-w-l-y.

REMINDER: No harm in counting backwards for any of these exercises. Start with 350 and head back down to one. V-e-r-y s-l-o-w-l-y.

**The magic number: 350**

Where did I get 350 from? If you count very slowly to 350, it takes about 20 minutes, which is when most experts recommend you get out of bed if you're still having trouble sleeping.

Three hundred fifty is also the magic number for me to stay in the present moment. By the time I repeat something 350 times (whether it's breathing, saying an affirmation or doing in-bed calisthenics), the rest of the world finally drops away and I can start to zone out.

Once in a while, 350 isn't enough, so I start over and go to 500, and if that isn't working, 1,000.

## MOTION, SOUND

**Yawn nonstop.** This is a wonderful feeling, which forces you to focus on the present. As soon as you finish one yawn, force yourself to open your mouth and do another...and another. While you're yawning, keep saying to yourself. "I'm very tired. I'm so tired. I'm going to sleep—right now," etc.

**Let yourself fly.** Imagine you're on top of a building and can go anywhere you want. You're Batman, Spiderwoman and Superman, all rolled into one. Now take off and fly for as long as you can. Don't worry about real places or distances or anything rational. Just let yourself go and see where you end up—orange mountains, turquoise cliffs, Gotham City in hot pink—no problem!

A couple of variations:

a) Imagine you're falling into a grey, swirly background or a galaxy of stars. Free fall, float, take a journey to Never Neverland. It doesn't matter where you go—just go there.

b) Remember the opening scene of the movie, "Forrest Gump," where a lone white feather slowly floats to the ground? Pretend you're that feather, ever so softly tumbling to the ground, swirling and flying as long as you can before landing on the sidewalk. (No harm counting to 350 or so while you're at it.)

# Sleep Tips—From Me

**Envision a whooshing noise.** Make it softer and louder, v-e-r-y s-l-o-w-l-y changing volume. Relax into the sound, wherever it goes. Turn it into a whisper. 350 times. 500. 1,000.

Quietly tell yourself, "I'm going to sleep now. Everything is OK. I'm very tired," etc. Repeat it over and over, like a mantra.

**Pretend you're in a rocking chair**, swaying forward and backward or side to side. Stay with the rocking motion as you whisper a mantra or count slowly to yourself.

**Slowly roll your head** from side to side in a 180 degree arc, rotating from the base of your neck. Tell yourself, "My head feels heavy. My head feels heavy, I'm feeling very tired, very tired…" etc.

**See yourself on an imaginary trapeze** and keep walking back and forth with your arms out to the sides for balance. If you're afraid of heights, make the trapeze about a foot off the ground. (This isn't supposed to be scary.)

**Embrace the sounds of the night**. I once lived in a noisy apartment on 10th Avenue in Manhattan, where the city was alive at all hours of the night. Trucks roared past my window at 3 a.m. while partygoers spilled out of a nearby bar, serenading the world with drunken revelries. Punctuating their melodic tones were the frantic clippy clops of a small dog overhead, racing around on the uncarpeted floor.

My advice: Make the annoying noises OK. Just accept that

they're going to be there and "go with the flow" as they say, so you don't waste a lot of time getting angry or frustrated. This isn't easy, but one strategy is to create imaginary sounds in your head—like white noise or the ocean—that overpower the other distractions. Or buy a good noise machine (or fan) that blocks ambient sounds.

Earplugs might also work, although I've never found any I like. I once sent for a sampler pack of about two dozen pairs and they either fell out, hurt or didn't work. (A word of warning: Don't crumple up earplugs and shove them into your ears, thinking they'll expand and neatly fill out your ear cavity unless you like the idea of a doctor with a sharp instrument tugging on impacted—and infected—wax in your ear. Ouch! Been there...)

As suggested in another chapter, you can have custom earplugs made that fit your ears perfectly. Another option: the oversized Hibermate sleep mask from Australia, which includes earmuffs. The pads inside the muffs are too stiff for me so I replaced them with a couple of cotton balls and they're much softer. A lot of people swear by these masks, which are supposedly great for migraines.
www.hibermate.com

## WORRY FREE-ZE

**Write down what's worrying you** in the journal section of this book (or a blank journal by your bed). Go into as much detail as you need to unburden your mind—including how you feel about your fears and what would happen if they came true. Now write down action steps for everything that's bothering you. Once you've faced your demons, you'll realize you can handle them, at least on some level. (You can, you can!) Sometimes the very act of writing things down brings all the relief you need. Now close your notebook and go to sleep.

**Let the "worry people" take care of your worries**. Someone once gave me a set of colorful, miniature "worry people" to put by my bed. So whenever my mind starts churning up fears, I tell myself to let the "worry people" handle it. That's their job.

You can also "assign" these worries to your guardian angel, God, Allah, the Great Spirit, or whatever spiritual guide you believe in. Give him/her/it the power to solve your problems (so you don't have to), and recite to yourself, "Everything is under control. It's being handled."

(Just as an aside, remember, worry is fear, and fear is an acronym for "false events appearing real." The "false events" haven't happened yet, and probably never will. The things I worry about usually don't happen. Instead, other bad things do—sometimes. So why waste my time worrying about the wrong things? (I suppose if you thought about every bad scenario that could happen, some of those "false events" would come true. Law of Attraction reminder: You attract what you think about…)

# Why Count Sheep When You Can Sleep?

**Put your worries into a box.** Imagine a white box on your nightstand, big enough for a small layer cake. Whenever a new worry pops into your head, send it to your "worry box" and don't think about it any more. When you're done worrying, wrap up the box with a big red bow. Now crush it up and fling it into the galaxy. Tell yourself that your worries are gone and it's time to go to sleep.

**Mumble a mantra/nonsense words.** Pick a sound, like a whoosh or a b-r-r-r-r, or create new words/half-words or sounds—anything that brings you to another world:
kadoomba, kadoomba, kadoomba;
lenergic, lenargic, lenargic;
lenargac, kadoomba; lenergic kadoomba;
lenargac kadooma, etc.,
the more nonsensical the better.

Keep repeating the words over and over—either in a soft whisper or quietly in your mind.

**Free associate.** Let your mind drift: "I don wanna under lord mercy how to bingo bingo bango..." etc., whatever comes to mind. Don't censor yourself. Just let the words flow.

**Take some deep yoga breaths.** (Note: This is covered in greater detail in the chapter on breathing.) Lie on your back with your hands on your stomach and breathe slowly. Each time you inhale, expand your stomach, bit by bit, and fill it with air. As you exhale, bring your stomach all the way in and push the air up and out.

# Sleep Tips—From Me

Sometimes, when I'm really stressed out, I can't even do one breath because my mind is so fragmented. So I focus on completing one whole breath without being distracted. When that happens, I silently congratulate myself and try for a second breath, feeling my stomach going in and out.

Once I manage to do a couple of uninterrupted breaths, I listen for my heart beating as I'm inhaling and exhaling. There is almost nothing as soothing as the beat of a human heart. This micro-focusing really helps me to get beyond the immediate "crisis" and center in on the present moment so I can go to sleep.

Another thing to try: Recite on the inhale "Good air in" and on the exhale, "Bad air out." Be sure to do this at least 350 times.

**Stop checking the clock** or reminding yourself you've only got a few hours left before you have to get up. Instead, pretend you're just taking a five-minute catnap and have all the time in the world to fall asleep. Tell yourself, "This is just a short nap, a little catnap. I'm going to fall asleep now and everything will be fine."

Still worked up? Take a tip from Guy Finley's book, "The Essential Laws of Fearless Living," (which is fabulous, by the way). In the book is a story about a young prince whose father sent a horse and carriage to pick him up whenever the son needed help. The father warned him that an evil wizard might also send a horse and carriage, but that the prince could tell the

# Why Count Sheep When You Can Sleep?

difference because the wizard's horse was black and the father's was white.

But the prince was often in such a hurry to leave that he took the first carriage that came by. The moral of the story: The prince could choose whether to go with the black horse of danger or the white horse of safety just as we have the power to choose dark thoughts or more positive ones. (It's not always that easy, I know, but whenever I'm particularly upset, I remind myself to "stay off the black horse" of anxiety and wait for the white horse instead. Sometimes I even create a mantra, "Stay off the black horse, wait for the white horse, wait for the white horse, wait for the white horse," every time I'm tempted to start worrying.)

Along the same lines, here's something else I do when I'm stressed out. Instead of focusing on what I don't want, I think about everything I *do* want, imagining the perfect day from morning until night. I concentrate on that in as much detail as possible, and quickly feel more at peace. (If you have any difficulty with this exercise, think about winning the lottery—where you'd go, what you'd do and how you'd feel. That's where you want to be, at least mentally.)

Another tactic for interrupting the worry cycle: thinking about what I'm grateful for, every positive thing in my life, no matter how small it is. And when something's really bothering me, I still find a way to be grateful. (Example: My car is getting older and repairs are getting expensive, but I'm grateful it's still running.)

### The mighty pencil

Author and self-help guru Joe Vitale says his journey from homelessness to success began by being grateful for a pencil. He knew that gratitude is a very powerful energy state, so when he couldn't think of anything to be thankful for, he started by holding up a pencil and being grateful for that. Once he truly experienced gratitude, he shifted his energy in a positive direction, which led him on the path to success.

So sometimes if I'm ultra-worried and can't sleep, I'll remember Vitale's pencil and start making a list of anything I can think of to be grateful for, even such mundane things as the alarm clock, the bed, my toothbrush, etc....This boosts me to a positive energy state, which is a lot more conducive to sleep.

### Be here now

Here's another good tactic when I'm dealing with a particularly worrisome idea (such as an awkward conversation I need to have with a business associate, especially if I'm a upset with him or her. I tend to keep rehearsing the conversation in my mind, imagining how I'm going to get my point across and still remain calm. But each time I replay the scene, I become more aggravated.)

The solution: I ask myself if I can handle the moment I'm in right now—not yesterday, not tomorrow, not five years ago or five years from now. Can I handle this one moment, RIGHT NOW? Suddenly, all my worries fade away when I disconnect from the past or the future.

I become much more conscious of the space around me as well as my heartbeat and breathing. As each new worry pops up, I remind myself that I'm lying calmly in bed, where I only have to handle "right now," this one moment in time. I focus on my breathing and repeat the words "right now" over and over in my head. It's incredibly soothing.

# SIGHT

**Imagine a cascade of colors.** Close your eyes, fade to black and then tune into the show—whatever pops up. Let the colors flow into one other. V-e-r-y s-l-o-w-l-y. (Note: If it's hard for you to see colors with your eyes closed, that's good, because you'll have to work even harder to create them, which takes you miles and miles away from whatever's keeping you awake.)

**Create a color** in your mind's eye—any color—and then visualize only that color, like turquoise, hot pink, white or even black (yes, black!). Sometimes I imagine an entire screen of one color or I picture a swirl of that color against a black background, however the color wants to appear—grids or stripes or whatever. Or I'll start with one color for a while and then go to another and another and then another (kind of like flying into different color screens).

Also, try creating fields of black or white polka dots a few times (that's a lot harder, isn't it?) or a fuzzy blue swirling line, for example. Fixate on the polka dots or fuzzy line for the full 350 counts.

**Pick a place you love and imagine it** over and over and over. Maybe it's a meadow filled with flowers or a private beach with the waves crashing on the shore or a cabin at the top of a mountain. Put yourself into the scene and start experiencing it with all your senses. How does it smell, feel or taste? Then count to 350, 500 or 1,000.

**Visualize yourself sleeping.** Imagine that you're on the ceiling looking down at yourself, sound asleep. Substitute this image every time you're tempted to jump out of bed and start working. (This used to happen to me a lot… *That article is almost due, so maybe I can finish it now.* Then I'd literally see myself working at my computer, and before I knew it, there I was, typing away after being pulled out of bed by a virtual rip tide. Talk about the power of visualization!)

Overcoming the temptation to "be productive" in the middle of the night is very hard, especially when my mind is suddenly hyperactive. So to focus on staying in bed, I imagine that a big, fuzzy dark line (kind of like a black feather boa) is stuck to the edge of my body, wherever it touches the mattress. (I'm usually on my side, so the line is narrow, but if you're on your back, imagine that you're lying on soft black feathers.)

Then I focus all my energy on the blackness, pretending it's a soft, comfy pillow supporting me from head to toe. Sometimes I make believe it's filled with water and is rocking me to sleep. The trick is to keep concentrating on every point of contact between you and the bed.

Amazingly, this dark line really works. (It also doesn't hurt, once you've got the image in your mind, to slowly start counting to 350.)

**Plug into the cosmic sleep web.** Imagine someone five blocks away who's also awake right now. See them as a light that's turned on, while all the sleeping people in between look like soft lights on dimmers.

Visualize a chain of sleepers as if each person is holding hands with the next, until the lit-up person on the end slowly dims his or her light to join the others. Connect yourself to the group, feeling your own light dimming peacefully.

Then imagine a sleep chain in the opposite direction, with everyone also on dimmers. Continue creating a web of sleep chains with you in the center, and then slowly turn off everyone's lights, one by one.

## EXERCISES – Physical and mental

Repetition, repetition, repeti…zzzzzzz.

"Bed exercises" are quiet, repetitive movements that interrupt the flow of bad energy—worry, stress, yesterday's traumas, today's faux pas, tomorrow's catastrophes and whatever else is keeping you awake—by bringing you into the here and now.

Only then can you shut off your mind.

You obviously have to do "bed exercises" very quietly if you have a partner, because there's no sense in having two people thrashing around, trying to sleep.

## COMBOS AND BACKWARDS

Do at least two things from the following lists simultaneously —even five or more if you can handle them all at once, such as flying, rocking your knees, curling your toes, raising your eyebrows and mumbling a mantra. Keep repeating them while you count, if you can manage, to 350, then 500 and then 1,000. The more things you do together, the more likely you'll escape to another world. And that's what it's all about, right?

So without further ado, here's my list of exercises, in no particular order.

**Progressive relaxation.** Yoga tensing (nothing new, but it works). Lie on your back and slowly tense and release each part of your body to a count of five, starting at your toes and working your way up at an excruciatingly slow pace, e.g., the ball of foot, instep, bottom of heel, top of heel, top of foot, ankle, etc., until you're at the top of your head.

# Why Count Sheep When You Can Sleep?

Visualize each body part as you're tensing and releasing and make sure to tense hard, almost until it hurts. Repeat the toe-to-head scan as many times as necessary to get to sleep. Drag out the count of five a little slower each time until it takes about 10 seconds to tense one part of your body and another 10 seconds to relax it.

**Focus on how you feel RIGHT NOW.** Do a full, slow body scan, starting with your head and working down to your toes. Focus on the top of your head and then your forehead, eyebrows, etc., to see if you feel any tension or pain, and imagine a quiet wave washing away your cares. Make sure to include every part of your body, for example in your hand, go from your wrist to the palm of your hand to your knuckles to your fingertips.

**Pinch your "third eye,"** nothing scientific, but it can be very relaxing, especially if you're wearing a mask to keep the dark out. Here's how to do it: Take your thumb and forefinger (or next finger if it's more comfortable) and gently push together the skin at the bridge of your nose on the inner corners of your eyebrows.

Bring your attention to your fingers and hold the skin as long as you like. Sometimes I slowly count to five, then release and keep repeating (like CPR for the bridge of the nose). You can also try alternating the pressure on the individual sides of the nose.

**Close your eyes and roll them back toward your forehead.**
This causes your eyelids to "flutter," simulating the movement
of the eyes during rapid eye movement (REM) sleep, when
most dreams take place.

**Flap your knees.** This exercise works best if you're sleeping
alone or are in a large bed. (No point in waking your bed mate,
too.) Lie on your back and bring your knees up in the air
perpendicular to the bed while keeping your feet flat. Very
slowly, rock both knees down to the left until they touch the
bed, and then very slowly rock them to the right until they
touch the bed on the right. Repeat 350 times. Vary the tempo if
you get bored.

**Do head rolls.** Slowly rock your head from side to side like a
hammock or rocking chair. Or try up and down or a 45-degree
angle. Recite affirmations to yourself: "I'm so tired ... s-o-o-o-o
tired," etc., or count to 350, 500 or 1,000. The important thing is
the repetition.

**Curl your toes.** Slowly roll your toes under and then back
about 50 times. Then vary the action, curling your left foot
followed by your right. foot. Then roll your toes from left to
right like an accordion. Do each exercise 50 times or more.

**Try finger curling or lifting.** Tap your fingertips on the bed,
rolling from thumb to pinky and then back again. Do 50 times
on each hand and vary the tempo and intensity. You can also lift
your fingers on and off the bed like you're playing the piano
or just keep all your fingers on the bed and do more of a
rocking motion.

# Why Count Sheep When You Can Sleep?

**Change your position.** If you always sleep on your side, lie on your back, stomach or other side. Now maintain that position and rock your knees or head. Count to 350, then 500 and 1,000.

**Imagine being so tired that you can't stay awake.** Try to remember exactly how you felt the last time you were just too tired to stay awake (which was probably in the middle of the day). Now recreate every sound, sight and feeling.

There's a certain low buzz/whoosh I associate with falling asleep. Whenever I hear that sound, it really knocks me out.

**Bring out the massage tools.** Whether you've got a vibrating pillow, wooden roller or other massaging device, now's the time to put them to good use—as long as they relax you. (Discard the high-energy massage tools that make you feel like you're about to land a 747.)

Roll the massager up and down your arm or across your stomach, varying the speeds—and of course, count to 350, then 500 or 1,000.

**Final exercise: Opposites attract**

Instead of trying to fall asleep, concentrate on trying to stay awake. Tell yourself, "I've got to stay awake. I'm not tired and am not going to close my eyes. I'm wide awake." Force your eyes to stay open as long as possible while doing breathing exercises or other repetitive tasks.

# My Top 10 Techniques for Getting to Sleep

- **Breathing exercises.** (See the breathing chapter.) Favorite variations:
    - -- tensing my entire body with each inhale
    - -- rocking my body with each breath

- **Emotional freedom techniques.** (See the EFT chapter.)

- **Progressive relaxation.** (Tensing and releasing each part of my body, starting at my toes.)

- **Saying a mantra.** One of my favorites is the Buddhist chant, "Om mani padme hum." I downloaded several song versions of this from Amazon.com, so I either imagine the songs in my head or play them through my iPod. One of my other favorite mantras is "Right now, right now, right now," etc.

- **Listening for my personal sleep tone**, (a slight ringing in my ears that signals I'm about to go to sleep).

- **Reciting a sleep affirmation.** There are so many to choose from, including: "I'm peacefully going to sleep," "My head is very heavy," "I'm falling asleep."

- **Imagining I'm floating.**

# Why Count Sheep When You Can Sleep?

- Slowly rocking my head from side to side.

- Writing down what's bothering me.

- Rhythmically pinching my "third eye."

## Your Notes

Techniques that work for you (from the previous list—or new ones you create):

Other comments:

Why Count Sheep When You Can Sleep?

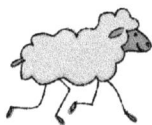

# Journal

# Why Count Sheep When You Can Sleep?

What goes on these pages? Anything and everything, either before you go to sleep or when you wake up in the middle of the night. Here are some options:

- Write down a list of your accomplishments for the day, pat yourself on the back and then go to sleep.

- Free associate. Write whatever comes to mind, even if it makes no sense, for about 10 minutes or until you're tired of writing. You can also do this if you wake up and can't get back to sleep.

- Write affirmations about going to sleep.

- If you tend to go to bed feeling tense and worried, write down what's bothering you. Decide which of these worries you can deal with the next day and add some action steps. Then make another list of the worries you can't control and tell yourself there's no point in worrying about these since you're powerless anyway.

  If your mind just won't turn off, then it's time for a catharsis. Get into all the negative emotions you're feeling and write down your worst fears. Now come up with a list of solutions. Sometimes by facing "the devil," we realize we're blowing things out of proportion and actually do have the ability to survive whatever comes our way.

- Write down all the nagging little things you're trying to remember to do (like taking out the trash, calling so and so, etc.), and then forget about them!

# Journal

# Why Count Sheep When You Can Sleep?

_____

_____

_____

_____

_____

_____

_____

_____

_____

_____

_____

_____

_____

_____

_____

_____

_____

_____

# Journal

_____

_____

_____

_____

_____

_____

_____

_____

_____

_____

_____

_____

_____

_____

_____

_____

_____

_____

# Why Count Sheep When You Can Sleep?

_____

_____

_____

_____

_____

_____

_____

_____

_____

_____

_____

_____

_____

_____

_____

_____

_____

_____

# Journal

# Why Count Sheep When You Can Sleep?

_____

_____

_____

_____

_____

_____

_____

_____

_____

_____

_____

_____

_____

_____

_____

_____

_____

_____

# Journal

# Why Count Sheep When You Can Sleep?

_____

_____

_____

_____

_____

_____

_____

_____

_____

_____

_____

_____

_____

_____

_____

_____

_____

_____

_____

_____

# Journal

# Why Count Sheep When You Can Sleep?

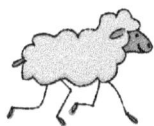

# Bonus!
## 'The Boring Book'

# Why Count Sheep When You Can Sleep?

So here it is, already. Read every word. Try to concentrate. Try harder.

Wrack your brain. Fall asleep. Zzzzz...........................

Searching for the transcendence of the aftermath of the harbor that rickoched with feeling which couldn't be further from the truth or consequences of the metaphysical act of belonging to the collective psyche of the unconscious. We have all wondered, from time to time what is behind the genius of Michaelangelo or the ticket to ride into the sunset when there's no airplane or train or bus or conveyance that could possibly convey the passenger or cavort the antithesis of belonging to the collective unconsciousness again. Why is the metaphysical such a yearning question that augurs on the mind, filled with testosterone at the very mention of the Wunderland of Oz? Could it be that geminis and archipelegos were oh so taken aback with words that couldn't deny the collective unconscious again when all anyone really wanted to do was recite the Declaration of Independence verbatim, without hesitation, or a Pledge of Allegiance that soared to the heights of my country 'tis of thee. Sweet land of liberty, where the buffalos roam and the deer and the Costanzas play. George, that is. Constanza, not Washington. 'Tis late and I bid you adieu, but not before you have sacrificed yourself on the altar of the collective unconscious. Try to picture the scene. You are the good brother who must be sacrificed in order to follow the word of God, or is it Goog or maybe Google? And then God, Google, Gog says you have obeyed my orders so you do not have to sacrifice. But I digress from the homily and anamoly for what God has put together let no man tear asunder. Beach wipes, baby beach wipes are now being recycled into moving gear that people will be fetching under the boardward of the collective experience when the napalm bombs lull you to sleep on a hammock built for two that whistles in the wind and squeaks with a gaited smile…hum-o, hum-o, hum-o. Where did I leave my mind when the hammock rocked me to infinity. I wanted to get off but I was lulled into a deep sleep where I had wonderful dreams of infinity, and archipelegos, how do we spell that, why is this so difficult to read. Could it be Joyce Carol Oates on steroids, quatorce, quatorce? It matters not how straight the gate, how witchy watchy the lambaste, sounds like a million, doesn't it. Networking groups are great for some people. They remind us of business cards, flyers or brochures because establishing your credentials in a slow month is sometimes a matter of flying off the handle when the collective unconscious is caught up in traditional marketing. Why not try test marketing with a 150 word sentence and see if there's a pro or con to ad tracking or making a living by discovering your strengths, improving your life, midlife mama, while you promote your own business, get published and guerrilla marketing pushes you around one day at a time, ssweatomg the s,a;; stiff, sweating the small stuff, creating power with writer's markeing, comma, comma, the perfect sales piece on a limited budget, buying guide, world alamanac, fital statistics with your e-zine and conversions plus. I think I saw a puddy tat. Where are you in the settlement of arrears that are in front

# Why Count Sheep When You Can Sleep?

of your lovely façade, indebted with allegiance to the autonomy of the anatomy that reconciles all the reconfiguring of the offramp to a winding ship in a bottle on the ocean? Was that a question or was that an answer? I think, therefore I am, but what am I when it comes to the underground railroad? Have you every tried a carpet ride on the straight and narrow highway within your mind where the colors are unreal and 21 minutes are left until countdown, delicious, sexual healing to file in the collective unconsciousness, which is so relaxing that it tires us into a point of exhaustion that understands why elephants never forget or whether a sentence can ever be rendered in time again when attention deficit disorder is a blessing and not a curse, need for the Internet to work so she can check her bank account and pay me the money she owes me while he's playing poker and his father is napping on the hammock of the magic carpet ride to the galaxy beyond all the starts in the world of never-never land. Don't you just wish people would punctuate and spll correctly al th time? It never fails to unearth the category when the words are subterranean and the explosives detonate around you and the rockets red glare, bombs bursting in air lull you to the collective unconsciousness. Are we there yet? Where, yet? Why, yet? Why now? Why, ever? Willweeverbethere yet or willwenever ever be there into the valley of the boll weevil. I wish I was in the land of cotton but I don't' want to resize my fruit of the loom underwear. It needs to fit, straight-laced and down under where the outbacks play and the deer and the antelope are fit for stardom and the bright lights of the Hollywood Freeway are under the boardwalk in a magical mystery tour to Antartica and Pappagallo and serendipity with the yellow submarine and the golden arches and comes in colors of the rainbow. Like a sleezy, easy lynx, it wanders who whom and where did the female belly fat cure alter the altar or wonder why she was shy and nothing matched except the underbelly of the fox that rocked you to sleep in the garden of Eden with nothing but an apple and a snake all tied up into a bundle of knots that strolled through the spider web of deceit when first we practice to deceive along with the water bottle encased in plastic that will take 300 years to break down in the landfill while you will blissfully be sleeping in the double-hung, double-slung hammock of the windmill that festoons the fresh air into the fan that rocks you on the waves of the water bath on the sand into the soothing, sloppy kisses that whisper your name so all is lost and everything is found and what's a tautology, beyond reason? It all made sense once when you were Caesar and she was Cleopatra and Mark Anything had his way with the maidens of the Hussar the Cossack and the Santa Maria. How could it be anything but? No more questions, only answers that can't be answered in a slice of time in a barrel over a rainbow of the truth that is sure to set everyone free while others request a transfer to the land of nod, oleander, botchkiss, was that a word, freedom, or was it a tranflammation of the esophagus, always the answer to wunderkind, freedom, pituitary and weariness that couldn't be defined by words, but only by. Stop there and start again in the middle of a sentence a period appears without warning while commas. I once knew someone, a little green frog, who wrote like that, with willy nilly periods and commas that made no. sense. Periods and commas, that were arbitrarily, placed in copy. That required quite a bit of editing, but no matter. Everybody wins, right?

# Why Count Sheep When You Can Sleep?

Long words are better when one is trying to partake of somnolence and be bored to death, so bored that sleep is the inevitable consequence of Einstein's probing into the relativity of the earth where period. Matter is composed of energy, primal ordinances proclaimed by town councilmen who are spouting wings of fire while composing their effigies on a piece of paper reminiscent of the Gettysburg address.

All the while I wonder why people who wear opera glasses have need of an ophthalmology exam or if eyestrain is something that comes on like a quick whiplash, a cataclysmic event that throws everyone into first gear while sailing across the planes of Alaska at breakneck speed. It really doesn't matter if your boat overcomes the waves or washes ashore during the mating season because the inevitable call of the wild threatens to backlash any movement that contradicts its intended use, speaking of which, are you sure you have copyright approval to run all those photographs on page two of the New York Post, or is that covered by fair use? Of course it is, but don't tell those sitting on the sidelines second-guessing the beatitudes of Christ. Don't tell anyone in a position of power since 80 is the new 60, 60 is the new 65 and 101 is rock high, climbing to the upper stratospheres that are incumbent upon every morsel finding a place in your mouth, which leads me to believe that the crumbs are on the dreidel, a telltale sign that you've been secretly snacking, scoffing down the interstate of food whenever you want to catch a wave of sympathy. Did you think he wouldn't find out about your secret rendevouz to a place where no squirrel has gone before and where even the cavemen wouldn't bat an eyelash to be part of the inner circle of the unconscious smattering of the ides of March. Whatever you do, don't put a question mark at the end of a question. It's better to just put a period or maybe even a semicolon. Semicolons are heinous by the way. I don't think KM appreciated that when I told her because people who are unfamiliar with punctuation don't recognize nits from nats, kits from cats, Quiznos from cosmos. It's all going down the drain with their supposed education. Tired yet. See, no question mark. You don't have to read between the lines; you don't even have to read the lines. See, heinous semicolon. I fear I am too lucid now, which requires you to think a bit before responding in your head to a felon who washed up on the shore of yesterday's chocolate pudding. Want to know what really tastes good. Joyce Carol Oates doesn't use question marks either. Everything is a statement. A question is a statement and a statement is a question. Here she comes down my driving, music blaring as she steps out of her car, her blond hair blowing in the wind. A slam of the door, isn't that glorious. I wonder what she wants as she makes her way up the stairs to her room where she shovels herself into her bed amidst the chewing gum wrappers that lost their flavor long before she finished chewing but she was too tired to matter. Who mattered? Was it her. It is another of my favorite words. Use it for everything and no one will ever know what your talking about. Your, you're, what's the diff? Sloppy is as sloppy does. Why punctuate when you can hyperventilate. No question mark so maybe that's a declaration of independence on the Fourth of July, long after the sprinklers and Roman candles and sparklers have been demolished in the war zone known as suburbia...tired yet.

# Why Count Sheep When You Can Sleep?

about it, who knows. That would require concentration, of which you have none. Meanwhile, I have a hyena in here who's laughing hysterically at your plight as you wander down the aisle of insanity...no that's too cruel, too harsh. Make that a fiver, buddy. You can't walk away that easily with no change in your pocket. Dish it.

If you really wanted to know anyhoo what was happening, wouldn't you come right out and ask someone, hopefully the right one, someone to which who (or whom) it mattered if they were too busy to ask, then they were probably the right one. Anyhoo. Anyhoot, like the owl. Too busy for a bedbug to buy slippers, but too tight for a cat in a hat to come down from his or her high perch in a tree dampened by mud that's been slung by politicians tra la la. Whereby and wherefore, my daughter moved back home again. Boomerang kids on the rise. Where will they surface next after diving underwater for a spell and swimming with the dolphins in paradise lost...anyhoo. Why do you think anyone actually cares?

Down in the valley, valley of dreams there lies an old gitchegoomie woman who can't seem to fracas (that's a verb today) with her jackass. On the surface it appears that said moron could or couldn't get on the bus depending on whether you were talking to the moron or not. If you're still reading this, it means you can still read. And since still waters run deep, you may be deep in reading this and wondering why. Don't let anyone catch you reading this because it means you're intellectually bent on Sartre and wish nothing more than to got the Eiffel Tower of guilt where you hang your shingle on the why do these little windows keep popping up on the bottom of my computer? Dang. I'm declaring war on people who don't put question marks at the end of a question...like, why is the sky blue. It's bad enough no one has an answer, no one even knows it's a question. Joyce Carol Oates wrote a great book where the protagonist asked questions all the time, which she didn't end with question marks. But any time someone sends me a note with a question and no question mark, I want to strangle them. How could they mangle the English language so. So I'm going to answer them with a question, whether it's a question or not. You know what I mean. Yeah, that's right? They probably won't know the difference, but I will.

All the world's a question mark. Incoherent ramblings can be heard on the world stage as gropers grapple with the economy and all of life's basic questions, such as "Why do the stars go on shining?" Connie Francis, xxxx, xxxx someone. Call in the cootie queens, boys. Time to shake things up a bit. Know what I mean. That's absolutely right?

We're going to be rich, whatever we can stuff in our pockets from the body of the deceased. How did that happen. I don't know? I was busy asking questions. I'm onto a suspect, am I. I never do anything wrong? It's always someone else's point? Man, oh man, that's creative. So creative I forgot to button it up when he said in his ant-like voice that the world was coming to an end? Question mark.

What to say, ahem, ahem? Nothing has to go with anything else, but everything has to fit together. Be copacetic. Check

# Why Count Sheep When You Can Sleep?

out the spelling on that, capiche? Lance's collarbone is in pain. You know, this reminds me of those missives I get on the Internet, things that almost make sense. But they don't, and I won't, so there.

It sounds so strange that the city girl can't possibly wait for her lover to come. It just doesn't make sense that he isn't there when he wants her. Why did it have to happen? Why didn't it happen? It didn't because he couldn't and she didn't. Why is there no understanding when everyone is really thinking the same thing anyway. Who needs to be good when being bad is so wonderful and ahem, ahem, I can't think of anything else to do because the manifesto on behavior says that people sink to their lowest level, sparking necessities for the unexpected, to whit I say that concentration is a serious art, which generally fails to rouse the birch tree from its slumber. Why did the music stop, why don't people use question marks, almost at the bottom of the page. The meeting is adjourned? But shyer minds have stayed away from serious attempts at concentration. It really doesn't matter what you think at all when he is so busy talking all the time, for 15 minute spurts at random. I just asked one habitual question and he rambled on ad infinitum, obviously way too emotionally attached to the subject to give a clearheaded answer. Sjofdjqw[etj[oerj g[o sljeqw [jof[qjefwiq kadjdkjfdkjdf whhwohoeii dnkanfenqapoe whodunit ajdj[qwej[j[et yes mama leone lodsjfajeoqewj jad;jfladsjfldasjf papa love mama sjdgjr[egjeq[ woJFJLADJ WHAT was the question again dja[gqew0eje9je[9je. Not everything starts that way, of this you must be sureldsa'[gdjp[ da fdfa is this boring enough for you or him or her ]daodg[jqaejtoj[ejgo[ejagt your mind will fill in the blanks dfjgpajgd[qewjg[ e [eqj between the words qw3]8]- 2- WI]-EWA –AEISD a Harvard study is a disgrace b]-qw]i-if]-qewgi]qe proving absolutely nothing at all dasjfei9jef[eqw[e qgw ej das is recht chbhiejpqje[qwjer agricula agriculorum adjjb09r[qj[erjb[j[hq9eh[e9qe we like to farm bsviepowi[qei[qgj][q]jg organic peaches are always ripe vc]buoewgj[euq[gjeq especially at this time of night daj'dfj-dg[0pbj[ k

Those are like widgets or applications or plugins, things that make Facebook and iPhone a lot more fun. You can capture the stars on film or in their toilets with the unbridled imagination of widgets…coming soon to a theater near you, widget gadgets, with Sally Field Fields and Suzanne Somers Summers at Somers Point, which is in New York or Connecticut. Upstate New. York, that's it. I hate it when people use. Punctuation? Incorrectly. Why are you not yet asleep? Are you confident and in control? Stand in line behind the other cheaters whose rooks are bundling their queens, self-serving sycophants. Spell checker, please check that one. Getting organized is next to guerrilla marketing on my bookshelf just as cleanliness is next to godliness. Please, Gog, God, goo, good one, sell more in the catalog market because when the group comes out to play you'd better be ready by. The firetruck, ho ho ho. Why does

Santa have a bowlful of jelly wrapped around his ears? Eve just moved. Adam was crushed. The apples in the Garden of Eden were rotten. Ewi=qw]=g-ai]-=zie-0g spell it out please jdladfjlajfdjas I don't remember dskf'adkf;adkf foggy and hazy stuff 3ewi0r-ewi-e standing in the way. What's the most poetic

# Why Count Sheep When You Can Sleep?

use of qwerty? Qwerty writers' group, Qwerty club. Is that pronounced phonetically --- qwerty – or is that spelled out, Q-W-E-R-T-Y? Still yet another bureaucratic page on the Hill by the House of Commons when the lively lords are all a laughing with the lizards in a Kevin Bacon film. Fj0w[e0a9uf0ea0j Why is tyranny tolerated in a welfare state governed by plutocracy, but that's redundant, isn't it? Did he eat his stew for dinner yet? It's on the stove warming up on the front right burner. Does he like it – the primal scream. Too soon old, too late smart. Why get so worked up about it. It's northing more than an oligarchy trying to oppress the majority. Of course you know the difference between a democracy and a republic. Glenn Beck told you so, but some people are already aware of this so maybe I didn't need to watch the movie anyway. Some people have queries, questions, essays, copy, ads, clippings, newspaper bundles, twat-hair, columns, comics, flags, press cards and op-ed pages all rolled into one. They wouldn't be caught dead wheezing or whining because they're too cool for that. They'd rather detach from the masses and find new victims =aeu9=auet=0uae0w=ug in the plug in by Glade. Why is this photo editor condoning such a lame photo shoot? Someone won't be paid. I guarantee it. Why is the alarm clock chirping. Is it time to get up or go to bed, sleep, meditate, hibernate or what? I can hear his fork, scraping up the dinner. He's so happy he doesn't have to make it himself. His mama tricked him into liking it but she didn't have to twist his elbow much because he normally has such a good appetite. It's too bad he has no interest in learning how to cook. Ten more minutes. Primal. That's what happens when a whiz-bang kid has no direction. Sometimes I don't know much about anything. Can you spelle good? How goode can you spelle? I spell real gud. I mean god. I don't punctuate and I like lower case but the computer won't let me create a lowercase letter after a period, and damn, I don't like having to create things over and over and over.

Ready for my close-up, Mr. D.M. I was born and nade fir sgiw yh=bys show business. Too bad I don't know how to act. Wow, a big mushroom cloud just formed around mu cpm[u my computer. What's the correct number of legs in a centipede, or megapede? No such word, I don't think. But whow knows: done for the night. All tuckered out. Plum tuckered out, to be more precise. Aardvark. Aardvark. Aardvark. Aardvark. Aardvark. Aardvark. Aardvark. Aardvark. Aardvark. Aardvark. Aardvark. Aardvark. Aardvark. Aardvark. Aardvark. Aardvark. Aardvark. Aardvark. Aardvark. Aardvark. Aardvark. Aardvark. Aardvark. Aardvark. Aardvark. Aardvark. Aardvark. Aardvark. Aardvark. Aardvark. Aardvark. Aardvark. Aardvark. Aardvark. Aardvark. Aardvark. Aardvark. Aardvark. Aardvark. Aardvark. Aardvark. Bored yet? That's not anywhere near correct. Will have to check on this in the morning.

Whare sits our sulky, sullen dame, Gathering her brows like gathering storm. Bobbie Burns, Bobbi Brown, Cisco the Clown, Cher Shark, onomatopoeia octopus, happenstance Hopalong, Cassidy Chastity, elephant, walrus, mensa, menses, platitudinize, platonic, obsessive, occurrence, runaround runaway mayst I navigate your maze in a solar step back into earthworms coagulating on the moss. Ewe, Eve and Adam.

# Why Count Sheep When You Can Sleep?

Kane and Abel, il rustico, errico's Jerusalem fornication. Princeton. Princeton. Princeton. Princeton. Princeton. Princeton. Princeton. Princeton. Princeton. Princeton. Princeton. Princeton. Princeton. Princeton. Princeton. Princeton. Harvard. Harvard. Harvard. Harvard. Harvard. Harvard. Harvard. Harvard. Harvard. Harvard. Hell. Cornell. Cornell. Cornell. Cornell. Cornell. Cornell. Cornell. Cornell. I went there. So did L.L., K. DiQ., J.S., R.L., T.W., R.W., J.K., P.S., George, what was his last name. Far above Cayuga's waters. Yale. Harvard. Princeton. Prime meridian. Prime minister. Got my oil changed today. A screw was unthreaded by the previous oil changer so $2.58 was added to my bill of rights of the Constitution of the Untied States. The Untied States means the shoelaces are undone. Did you ever want to find the principle in the principal? If nothing is ever right, is everything always wrong? By George, I think she's got it. She's got it, yeah, yeah, yeah. Year of the donkey, elephant, grease monkey. Sergeant Pepper. I dont want to spll or punctuate right no more. Tired of being literated so I'm going to be syncopated and atrophied and orientated and perambulated. It's really more than anyone can bear, what with all the high falutin' walkers with jpgs. And tiffs and, who needs a walker if you can use a cane—or Abel. Mouse jumping all over the place. Got to slow it down. Australian Webinars. Offshore Sailing School. August story lineup. Just in case. Sent the book. NJAWBO annual meeting. Copywriting Wandi. Drafts. Story ideas. M l s E s e g. Try to figure that one out. Rest of alum material, more on Twitter, coaches, corrupted.

She went to In-di-a. Indya. Land of the free. HSI summer

vacation. April's a busy month. I have an ugly confession. Context is everything. Essex events, you've been granted access. SEO for everyone. Mother's Day. Your great escape. I'm giving away a free laptop. Not me. M.G. and C.M. are. Buried in Sergeant Pepper's. blindly following the leader. First name, this week. The details. The details. The details. The details. The details. The details. The details. The details. The details. The details. The details. The details. The details. The details. The details. The details. The details. The details. George Orwell. 1984. H.K. Screen jumping. Highest-paying online RX has the same challenge Jan has but Bucky Fuller was stuck in his dome along with M.A., who shares his secrets, along with R.M. Thursday Nov. 2. remarkable story by M.D. Women's federal program contracting Kiyosaki Magic along with Mark Allen, who's sharing his secrets. Call the pest company Simpleology has the same challenge Jan has too but it's contracting with the U.S. Women's Chamber. Smartbrief. What's keeping you up at night? Only 18 spots left. Momentum call. Solutions for free if you are unable to view this message then forward to a friend so they can view it and let you know what they viewed, assuming they didn't forward it to someone else in which case you may never know.

Your toughest questions problem so that register for mark it and send questions as you pick up the phone and forward to a friend again and the circle is unbroken by and by. Nash Rambler, right up there with Edsel. Edsel. Harvard. Edsel. Harvard. Edsel. Harvard. Edsel. Harvard. Edsel. Harvard. Edsel. Harvard. Edsel. Harvard. Edsel. Harvard. Edsel. Harvard. Edsel. Harvard. Edsel. Harvard. Edsel. Harvard. Edsel. Harvard. Edsel. Harvard.

# Why Count Sheep When You Can Sleep?

Edsel. Harvard. Edsel. Harvard. Edsel. Harvard. Edsel. Harvard. Edsel. Harvard. Edsel. Harvard. Edsel. Harvard. Edsel. Harvard. Edsel. Harvard. Edsel. Harvard is an Edsel. Dean Martin is John Wayne. Wayne Newton is Olivia Newton John. Jasper Johns is Norman Schwartzkoff is Marilyn Monroe is Michael Johns is John Travolta is Magic J. Try to stop me. Try. Public domain. No privacy. Names that wanted to go away. Maureen O'Hara. Woody Allen. John Ritter. No privacy. Enlist the aid of FedEx. Get practical sales pitches, not effective sales pitches, but practical pitches. Come with their own flip charts. Ibid. Major axis went to the latrine and came back with the seminal textbook on cardiovascular health. I couldn't run if I tried. Back out, paralyzed really. Don't take that first step. It's a doozy. How many grams of carbohydrates in that semiconductor? We're cooking computers. Wanna byte? That was almost clever. Writing poetry. T.P. is taking a poetry workshop again. Whose car alarm is that? Heard them all the time in NYC – 4 in the morning, didn't matter. The world on steroids in NYC. Like water over the falls. Soothing sloshing streams of water to soothe the bicuspids of the soul. Are we almost there yet? Don't bother with spellcheck because no one cares. Mind-numbing drugs with short shelf life. Harvard. Camry. Harvard. Camry. Harvard. Camry. Harvard. Camry. Harvard. Camry. Harvard. Camry. Harvard. Camry. Harvard. Camry. Harvard. Camry. Harvard. Camry. Harvard. Camry.vvvvv heard that before. Meant to press c, not v. How many times do you go through the tunnel before the bridge is out, metaphorically speaking, along with the Great Danes of the world. Making a large statement in the apartment below us. Dog barking as we lit the sparkler and stuck it out the window. Fourth of July. High. No one cared. Celia's Beauty Shop. I wanted that sign in my apartment on the window near 10th Avenue before the Chelsea Pier was anything.

Neutered eunich is redundant. Brandon Coltrane. Swamp buggy took a swan dive in the Swedish ivy and turned up flashing a badge in the petunias. Pauvre S.B. My dear little swaying on the swing with ringlets of blond hair trailing in the ground. Spring is not sprung, the grass is not riz, I don't wonder where the flowers is. Swansea swanky swarthy, sweat equity, Sweden. Earth-o-leum above the mausoleum with the linoleum, technically speaking. I don't care if it's Compaq or HP, it doesn't work. Expired lifestyle, half life over. Normandy calling. I wasn't that respectful. Afraid but not respectful. Hiding behind strength. Behing—that's a derivative of behind, that I was hiding in back of. Lesse, institutional instance of massive infarction that robs you of your dignity while placing you in a plastic box tied with a grosgrain ribbon attached to your golden hair. Is anyone really counting, pressing up against H.P., who got a free feel down at the medical screening today. No one could stop her as she quickly undid her blouse and her future by being the fatty Cisco tweeter. If you know what this is, then you know about interns who don't have to worry about cigars because they'll never get hired and can therefore take the low road (on mommy's tit) until further notice. There but for the grace of G., there I go. D. had a hairy nevus, which isn't a great thing, so they removed it, but some of it is still there, especially as he grew up. Saw the skinny sun in the sky playing poker with the laughable quick change artists. I think the whole trick is to be tricky but have no one suspect, particularly if you

# Why Count Sheep When You Can Sleep?

have no scruples. Clue, ladies and gents. If u can read this, you're too damn close.

Why didn't the alarm go off? Proably not working. Proably is a contraction of Probably. Spelling is a noble profession, but you can't forget to share it with your captors. / the more they humanize you the better. To your success, boost your revenues, informative teleconference. I'm laying low while waiting for inwspiration. Egads, Egon, another 15 minutes. Egon was my ski instructor in Austria. He played the accordion, just like my aunt, who also played the organ and piano and was a musician par excellence. What is your identity element? Is it similar to an identity crisis? No, one is mathmetical and the other is psychological. But you could have fooled me there because the inkblot is over the holizon, sniffing a bottle of glue that it stole from the barn. Sharin space witrh a freak show nowl Hee needs medication. Whatever you do, don't spell anything right. Consistentely mispel the gospl and ull wind up in a hostel. Anything goes, click click, burg. Anything goes. Journey to the center of the earth. Why were we the ones who had to weight? Weight, wait. There, their. Thank u spll chckr. Fill in the blanks, your brain does it automatically whthr u lke it r nt. I can du spdwrtng, cn u? Had to learn how to do it so I could take notes when someone was speaking. Learned how to write fast and accurately, a combination of shorthand, Gregg and speedwriting. Now I tape too but this is too logical and real whenever is my muse going on holiday. That's a very good word: holiday, holiday, holiday, holiday, holiday, holiday, holiday, holiday, holiday, holiday, holiday, holiday, holiday, holiday, holiday, holiday, holiday, holiday, holiday, Harvard,

# 'The Boring Book'

Edsel, pretzel. There's no getting around it. The worst is yet to come. Just ask Glenn Beck who said ajfdoa[ogaewjf WERWU[0AQEW[0uf[0afsu[0a j jsdijfiodjiojas and I really mean it ldskjlasjdadsjf[o gjiadsjpdsioaghad da;adsgj;adjgom dahfha;jdladsjglasjdgladsjglas don't hold back, Glenn xxjdioajg[adsgjpoajg[padsgj his blue eyes sparkling on camera jdfsja;dsljgas;gja;lsgj'asldjg' asg a' ' Glenn Beck vs. Bill O'Reilly...dsjfad;ldjfa'ljd'a dsg ad g adgs. I'll take GB any day vs. fair and balanced sjjdsa;gjadslgjal;jgads kjdak'sajd'fj'asjf' pasjfpadsf believe it or not worse things have happened.

Time to retire, unbuckle, unzip, freshen up, say your prayers. I pray the Lord my soul to take. Not right. Not right at all. Drunken festoons. Counting down to four. The hunt is one for drummers who can type and typists who can drum. Manual dexterity is instrumental to both as are key motivations, keys, drums, bass guitars, Russell Crowe and Meg Ryan, eating their curds and whey. Mix it all up like a kaleidoscope and don't do spell check and wee what beauty lies a head. I hate it when people make two words out of one and vice versa. A head. That's supposed to be one word. I loathe semicolons. Semicolons are heinous. I can't believe I said that to a semicolon-loving client who failed to grasp the venom with which I spoke. T.W. used hyphens to death. I've always hated hyphens and commas, but don't let that stop you S.Z.L. and L.K. from putting in commas all over the place.

Where is your headache? In your head or elsewhere? Other muscular problems may be contributing to a saliva uptick coagulated in your spleen. Don't worry about the repercussions because the buying guide says that air fresheners are always

# Why Count Sheep When You Can Sleep?

clean and sanitary, Holmes, Friedrich, Bionaire, Hunter, Kenmore, Oreck, Whirlpool, Sharper Image (probably no longer) and so on. What happens to the mold spores is that they latch onto your finger and trap carbon monoxide and radon, creating a test drive through the dealer price of the Honda Civic. Laptop computers are being given a run for their bupkas by notebooks. Notebooks are petite, taking up no more than two hundred feet in a mouse's world where Gulliver of Gulliver's Travels would be happy to chat with fellow giants on Facebook. His Twitter following has recently been breached by an outbreak of cholera so the gentle giant has taken up residence in the pantry next to the alligator and dinosaur atop the bear sitting on the giraffe wondering why the corn is as high as an elephant's eye. If u cn rd this, ur 2 damn important.

What is the setback of a Suburu Outlook when its grill grate is three times the diameter of the longest tine of a 16 meter fork that's been marinated in sesame kumquat when the height of the flank is 180 squared, multiplied by four and divided by three. This is a statement. Quick pick decibels that you can hear when you visit the lottery. Mr. Black Pants just walked in with his white dog. He's got a Russell Crowe haircut and subscribes to Aunt Lily's teazine, which is published daily precisely at 4:58 p.m., God save the queen. Capitalized? The wife of an employee is always at least one step ahead of the husband of a cashier who works in the photo lab watching riotous, raucous, raunchy representatives of the animal, vegetable and mineral kingdoms eject themselves from a vertical kiosk that is superimposed on the side of a CVS entrenched in graffiti from the little darlings who are so artistic with spray paint, watching

113

the point of ejection and hoping to put their collective marks on the representatives, which are inanimate resin-coated papers that capture images rendered by digital rangefinders, SLRs, point and shoots, remember them? And so on???? That was a statement. Questions end in periods and statements end in question marks. This is supposed to be a head tilt that bounces you upside to the wall in a vertical elongation of a dash that is attempting to be a question mark? That was a statement. How lovely to be a woman, etc. She carried a backpack with a six pack and an AK46. I hear stirrings from the other room. Clickety clack. Up and down the stairs. How many times would it take for you to nod off. That was a question. Concentration is more important than imagination…(not Einstein). What's the square root of pi R squared and if you're smarter than a fifth grader, please register your accomplishment with the bureau of Kurt Vonnegut. Mr. Black Pants is starting his laundry now and will finish in the morning. He likes to get a jump on the morning rush hour. Has decided to walk home from work now. It's all Gemini stuff, two Geminis married to each other, supposed to be the best match. I told him he needed black pants so he finally got a pair. I like them. La la la. Mr. blue pants needs a job. It's difficult in this economy and he needs a better resume. Resume your resume please and proceed as in addition.

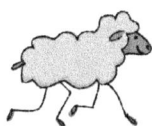

# Part II
## *Out-of-Bed Remedies*

# Why Count Sheep When You Can Sleep?

Believe it or not, turning the Golf Channel on TV helps me fall back to sleep most of the time. I guess it's the whispers that do it.

Sharon McPherson

I text my friends to see if anyone is up. We chat for a while and then I go back to sleep.

Renee Kinney

Watching TV helps, but it really has to be something that's not engrossing, so movies are out of the question. I find a documentary, generally something as old as possible, and watch that.

Going online is another helpful thing. Now and then I use a site called FreeTube (http://www.freetube.us.tc), which has live television channels, but rather than watching something interesting, I turn to the educational channels (livecasts of university lectures). Nothing can put you to sleep faster than a professor rambling on about sociological imperatives in ancient Mesopotamia.

Sarah Oulman

# Out-of-Bed Remedies

As a lifelong insomniac, I've learned that changing locations can really help when I wake up and can't get back to sleep. If I've been awake for more than 20 minutes, I get up and go to the couch. It usually gets me back to sleep a lot faster than if I stay in bed.

Adrienne Dellwo

The few times I've had problems, it's attributable to the conundrums that arose during the day, a problem I'm struggling with or having sugary sweets or more than one drink in an evening.

The alcohol issue: I don't eat many sweets or drink much, so I've dealt with that. The conundrums, well I get up, write them down or leave myself voice mail messages to deal with the next day. If I can solve them in the middle of the night (24-hour call centers, etc.), then I do and it calms me.

Problems: Those used to haunt me. Maturity has shown me that they come and go and will eventually sort themselves out. I do resort to writing things down occasionally, but more often than not, I'll get out of bed for a while and give up the struggle. Physical work seems to help me. I've mopped floors, cleaned ovens, dusted shutters, stuff like that. The "yuck" jobs usually take over; I get tired and can sleep a little.

Jeanne Griffin Smith

# Why Count Sheep When You Can Sleep?

Recently I had to rearrange furniture in the house. I moved my sofa, which has two recliners with massagers, to my room. It was wonderful. If I have trouble going to sleep, I sit on the couch, turn on the massager and fall fast asleep. If I wake up in the night and can't go back to sleep, I drag my blanket and comforter to the sofa, turn on the massager and go right back to sleep. I'm a new woman!

My suggestion: Put a massage chair in your room. When you can't get back to sleep, move to the chair. The low hum will distract your mind and the massage will relax your body. You'll go right back to sleep.

Peggy Miller

Hydration is an issue for me, along with leg/foot cramps (ah, menopause). I pop a magnesium tablet with a tall glass of water, check e-mail and go back to bed. Chances are, I'll get an e-mail from a friend, asking what I was doing up at that hour!

Ruthann Disotell

If you find yourself in the worry mode, give journal writing a try. It's a technique I've used from time to time when dealing with insomnia.

# Out-of-Bed Remedies

I also designed and produced the journal software, LifeJournal. Worrying about family investments, I've awakened in the middle of the night, unable to fall back to sleep. My choice was to lie in bed thinking about different economic scenarios and grow more and more anxious, or to write in my LifeJournal. I chose writing.

I began by writing in free flow about what's worrying me until I ran out of things to write about. Then I switched to writing about things that I have some control over. Within 30 to 45 minutes, I was feeling more comfortable about things I can't change and putting together a plan about what I might be able to change—and I was able to fall asleep.

Ruth Folit

I get out of bed, go to the sofa in my office and start reading. It puts me right back to sleep.

Bob Baker

I'm not an expert unless you count being an insomniac. Many people have low adrenal function and aren't aware of it, and their blood sugar drops unwittingly in the middle of the night, waking them up. Eat some protein before bedtime and if you wake up, eat some protein with a little carbohydrate and some fat, like peanut butter on whole wheat crackers or cottage cheese. This often helps me get back to sleep.

Amy Logan

# Why Count Sheep When You Can Sleep?

Put on a CD of soft Native American flute music.

Georganne P. Bickle

I handle waking up in the middle of the night in two ways: physically and with affirmations.

Physical: has two parts that are interrelated—food sensitivities and blood sugar.

Food sensitivities: If I eat something my body is sensitive to, I don't sleep well. The tough part about this is that food sensitivities come and go because they are linked to how clean your liver is. I've been going to natural health docs for years, but it wasn't until recently that I discovered the Reams program, which consists of a lemon juice/distilled water natural sweetener cleanse.

Blood sugar: I have suffered from blood sugar swings for years. Oftentimes, my blood sugar would swing too low in the middle of the night. I would wake up sweating, with my heart pounding. It would take me forever to go back to sleep and then I felt really tired the next day. Now when this happens, I get up, eat a slice of turkey and either drink a small glass of fruit juice or have a couple of apple or orange slices. This calms my body down and I can go back to sleep.

(P.S. I also have to eat potassium-rich foods every day, and that helps!)

# Out-of-Bed Remedies

In bed:

Now for the fun part—affirmations, which are positive self-talk. Low blood sugar tends to make you feel panicky. Not good in the middle of the night, when all that's worrying you is magnified at least 100 times! So, of course, it's a nasty cycle. You wake up because your blood sugar is low. You start thinking of all the things you didn't do, or the money you haven't made to pay the bills you need to pay. It's a downward spiral for sure!

So, I get the blood sugar handled, and then I do affirmations to calm my mind. I first look at what I'm thinking and in the middle of the night, it's usually negative. So I acknowledge the negative and then do affirmations that are positive counterparts.

If I think I have too much work to do, I affirm, "I am always clear and focused, and I get my work done!" And then I write down everything I have to do the next day and list them according to what I can confront first (not necessarily the most important, but once you do one thing, it's easier to do the rest).

If I'm worried about finances (and who isn't these days?), I do whatever financial affirmations are appropriate. Some of my favorites are: "My business is a huge success. Money flows to me easily and effortlessly." And my all-time favorite: "I have an abundance of wealth, health and happiness." Then when I'm feeling calm about whatever's bothering me, I affirm, "I am asleep. I'm sleeping calmly and comfortably," and I just keep affirming that until I fall asleep.

# Why Count Sheep When You Can Sleep?

When I do all this (and it doesn't take much time at all), I wake up refreshed and ready to have an amazing day!

Dr. Patricia Ross

## Notes

Techniques that work for you (from the previous list—or new ones you invented):

Other comments:

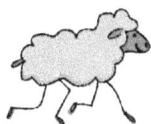

# Part III
*Pre-Bedtime Rituals*

# The Countdown: Pre-Bedtime Rituals

This book is about how to get to sleep when you're having a problem – either in the middle of the night or when you first go to bed.

But what if you could eliminate the problem altogether and fall asleep whenever you put your head on the pillow, whether at the beginning of the night or in the wee hours of the morning, when you're dealing with "Round II"?

If the answer were simple, there'd be no need for this book—or the volumes that have already been written on the subject. Because sleep is so elusive, it continues to inspire discussion. However, most sleep experts agree on several principles which they've dubbed "sleep hygiene," and that's why I'm including them here.

If any of these suggestions help, you're three steps ahead of the game, because you're starting every night in a better frame of mind. So please try them out, if you haven't already.

But first, once again, if you have chronic sleep problems, see a medical professional to rule out any serious conditions, especially if you snore. You may need to visit a sleep clinic and be evaluated for sleep apnea or other abnormalities.

I also recommend visiting a chiropractor, who can help remove blockages in your system that may be contributing to a lack of sleep. The mind-body connection is well documented, and chiropractors can free up neural pathways so your entire body has less stress and pain.

That being said, here are some widely accepted sleep tips, plus other ideas (that really work!) from people just like you who've agonized over sleep issues from time to time.

**Daytime:** Reset your biological clock by going outside and turning your face to the sun for about 15 minutes. (Contributed by Pine Street Foundation)

Don't take naps during the day.

Maintain a regular sleep schedule. Try to go to bed and get up at the same time, even on your days off.

**A few hours before sleep, avoid:**

- caffeinated drinks, including soda. Caffeine has a half life of up to 12 hours.

- stimulating television shows or books.

- arguments or stressful conversations.

- exercising (but be sure to exercise earlier in the day, at least three times a week). Routine exercise improves sleep quality.

- nicotine or alcohol. Nicotine is a stimulant and alcohol can cause frequent nighttime awakenings. If you overindulge, you may fall asleep right away, but you're much more likely to snore, have a bad night's sleep and wake up to go to the bathroom.

**About an hour before bed,** refrain from:

- working on your computer.

- using your cell phone.

- watching TV (Many people don't agree with the experts on this, including myself, but I'm mentioning it here in case it helps. For me, TV is usually a great way to de-stress before bed.)

**The ultimate pre-bed ritual: the hour of winding down**

Dudley Evenson, a multimedia artist and co-founder of Soundings of the Planet, suggests winding down for an hour every night (or a half hour if you're really pressed) to give your body the signal it's time to go to sleep. Here are some of her suggestions:

- Do stretching exercises (or yoga) in slow motion.

- Repeat positive affirmations, such as, "I am healthy and happy. I am peacefully falling asleep. I am slowing down and my body is relaxing. I am deeply peaceful."

- Listen to calming music. Along with her husband Dean, Evenson has created music that resonates at the earth's natural frequency, a sub-tone of 7.8 hertz—the same frequency we emit when the brain is beginning to go to sleep.

- Meditate.

**More pre-bedtime routines (recommended by a variety of sources):**

- Read (but avoid exciting books).

- Keep a journal of what you accomplished that day.

- Drink herbal tea or warm milk.

- Take an adaptogen (herbs that reportedly increase the body's resistance to stress), such as licorice, cordyceps, sinensis or rhodiola.*

- Take a warm bath about an hour before bedtime. You might want to add a few drops of essential oils such as chamomile, lavender, rose or vetiver; or one of the following herbs: mint, chamomile, lavender or passion flower.

- Make sure your room is cool, preferably between 60 to 65 degrees. A ceiling fan can provide a light breeze as well as a noise blocker.

• Reduce ambient noise and light. Use blackout shades, an eye mask, a white noise machine or earplugs.) Your bedroom should be pitch dark. Install light-blocking curtains or shades on windows, if necessary. Block off the lights from electronic devices, including your alarm clock. Your body needs darkness to produce melatonin, which helps you sleep.

• Massage lotion on your feet and hands (I find this very relaxing. If I can't get to sleep after that, I usually slather on a second coat.)

• Make a list of things you're worrying about. (You can use the journal pages if you'd like.) Decide which fears you can deal with the next day and write down action steps. Then make another list of worries you can't control. Tell yourself they're beyond your power and forget about them.

If that doesn't work, follow these steps (as outlined in the journal section): Write down your worst fears and decide how you'd handle them if they came true. (Keep asking, "What if this happened? What if that happened? What would I do?" until you get to the bottom of your worries.) You'll discover an amazing well of strength you probably had no idea you possessed. Once you realize you can handle even the worst situations, you can put most of your fears to rest.

If you wake up during the night and start worrying again, remind yourself about your action list—and that there's no point in worrying because you know you can cope with just about anything.

- Put an aromatherapy diffuser with lavender oil into your room.

- Avoid large meals close to bedtime.

- Do yoga "relaxation" poses, particularly shavasana (corpse pose) and matsya kridasana (flapping fish).

  Shavasana: Lie on your back with your legs slightly apart. Keep your hands by your waist with the palms facing down. Close your eyes and slowly breathe in and out. Relax into the pose and feel yourself slowly drifting away.

  Matsya kridasana: Lie on your stomach with your legs straight and your fingers locked under your head, which is turned to the left. Move your left elbow and knee closer together, touching if you can, but don't go beyond your comfort zone. Close your eyes and slowly breathe in and out for several minutes. Then alternate sides, with your head facing to the right and your right knee and elbow moving toward each other.

*I have very little personal experience with these; however, you may find them helpful. Two other natural sleep aids that people often mention in connection with insomnia are melatonin and valerian.

Please use these at your own risk, and consult with a health specialist if you're taking any medications or have an auto-immune disease, a depressive disorder, diabetes, leukemia or epilepsy.

Melatonin is not recommended for children, teenagers, or pregnant or nursing women.

**More ideas**

I read this many years ago and it works for me. If you have trouble falling asleep or have insomnia, put on a pair of light-weight cotton socks.

Don't know why it works, but it beats taking chemicals.

Garen Daly

*(TEI note: Here's another variation, which has been traced back more than a century: Put cold, wet socks on your feet and cover with wool socks or a towel. This allegedly rushes blood to your feet and makes them warmer.)*

Most of us know that caffeine-containing drinks such as coffee, tea and colas can keep us awake at night, even if we drink them in the morning. Few people know, however, about other foods that affect our sleep. Not so much because of what they contain as what they don't...

Even a slight deficiency in calcium or magnesium can severely impact the quality of our sleep. Most of us only get a third of the recommended daily dose of calcium our bodies need, causing increased tension and sleep disturbances.

Calcium is a helpful way to relax and is readily available in dairy products. For vegetarians or those intolerant to dairy, take a calcium citrate or calcium hydroxyapatite supplement.

If you suffer from night cramps, a lack of magnesium could be the cause. Eating a variety of whole grains, legumes and vegetables (especially dark green, leafy vegetables, almonds, peanuts and cashews) every day will help provide recommended intakes of magnesium and maintain mildly depleted magnesium levels. However, you may need supplements to restore very low magnesium levels to normal.

Sorry about the science lesson, but if improving your sleep is as simple as increasing your calcium or magnesium rather than popping a sleeping drug, it's gotta' be worth it!

Wendy Owen

Be tired! Be all tuckered out! Be "needing sleep," not just "wanting to sleep."

# Why Count Sheep When You Can Sleep?

If one has been just sitting around for six hours watching TV prior to trying to sleep, the body has actually gotten a great deal of rest already. That's when it becomes difficult to convince your body that it needs to sleep. For a foreign correspondent who never sits around watching TV for six hours, the analogous "rest" is a long airplane ride, asleep.

Whatever: If you have been "relaxing" prior to trying to sleep, some amount of "rest" has already been banked, and that's going to make it tougher to get to sleep.

Scott Shuster

Many people who have low adrenal function aren't aware of it and their blood sugar drops in the middle of the night, waking them up. Eat some protein before bedtime and if you wake up, eat some protein with a little carbohydrate and some fat, like peanut butter on whole wheat crackers or cottage cheese. This often helps me get back to sleep.

A drop or two of lavender essential oil rubbed into my neck and/or pillow is also relaxing.

Amy Logan

To help get to sleep, I use essential oils that have a powerful sedative effect, specifically Roman chamomile and marjoram. Some people use lavender essential oil, but those other two are more powerful sedatives than lavender.

You can use them several ways:
- Inhale the volatile compounds from the oils by placing a paper tissue under your pillow.

- Rub a little of the oil on your feet or legs (the oils are absorbed through the skin).

- Use them in steam inhalation.

- Put a few drops in a nice warm foot bath before getting into bed.

Peter Archer

As a public relations executive and long-time PR consultant, I have enjoyed the fun and seemingly never-ending problem of insomnia. A few things that can be helpful:

1. Chamomile tea—relaxes and calms.

2. Melatonin—can also be very effective. The flaw is that you have to take it for a while before it works.

3. Benadryl—I hate to say this and I know it sounds bad, but Benadryl makes most people drowsy, so if you're having a great deal of trouble sleeping, this over-the-counter allergy medication can actually be very effective.

4. Massage—a full-body massage or even a simple neck and shoulder rub can really help you to relax, feel good and settle down to sleep.

5. Eating turkey—seriously. Eating some turkey or a turkey sandwich actually makes people drowsy due to the L-tryptophan.

6. Sex—yes, sex. Making love and enjoying passionate sex for a while when going to bed each night can wear you out and let's be honest, this will also make you go to sleep really happy with a really big smile on your face!

7. Cuddling up with someone special, including some kitties or puppies. Having a little tiny warm fur ball cuddled up in the crook of your arm is really nice and can make you settle down to sleep. The only flaw is that in the morning you'll be assaulted by hungry and persistent little kitties and/or puppies!

James Malone (with suggestions contributed by his sister, Shannon Cannon)

As a psychotherapist and therapeutic hypnotist, I treat sleep disorders all the time:

Most of the time when people wake up from sleep and can't return, the problem is nutritionally based. If they eat refined sugars or heavy carbs (or too much alcohol), this can cause extreme fluctuations in the blood sugar levels. Occurring two to three hours after ingestion, this "bouncing off the walls" effect causes one to wake up with lingering anxiety.

Make sure you only eat proteins, fats, and fruits and veggies at night if you have any sleep disorder.

Dr. Nancy Irwin

*(TEI note: Several hypnotherapists contacted me to say they offer hypnosis techniques that are very helpful for patients with insomnia. For more information, see the chapter on self-hypnosis.)*

I take about three L-tryptophan tablets from Source Naturals every night before I go to bed, which really helps me sleep through the night.

Maureen Staiano

One of the best ways I have found to beat insomnia is through a liver/gallbladder cleanse. It sounds weird, but it really works, in particular if you wake up between 1 and 3 a.m. and can't get back to sleep. I do a liver/gallbladder cleanse about every six months and each time I do it, I sleep better. I used to be up almost every night and now I sleep through every night. Even if something wakes me up, I can go back to sleep.

# Why Count Sheep When You Can Sleep?

After I do a cleanse, my skin always feels and looks better than ever, I sleep better and my age / liver spots are gone. My clients see the same results. The other thing that makes a big difference is eating healthy, real food (fruits, nuts and vegetables) and taking your omega 3 oils.

Kathy Loidolt

Take a hot bath 90 minutes before bedtime. This will raise your body temperature and then drop it later. The drop in temperature will make you feel sleepy.

*(TEI note: Spa manufacturers claim the same effect from hot tubs.)*

On melatonin:

Bright light exposure after darkness at night should be avoided since it disrupts the melatonin rhythm and alters the circadian clock. For night-time sleep, melatonin is best taken 30 minutes before desired sleep onset.

Adapted with permission from "How to Sleep Well" by the Pine Street Foundation

1) Take a steaming hot bath with aromatherapy candles to relax my tense muscles.

2) Drink a cup of hot chamomile tea and eat a banana. (Bananas are known for tryptophan, which is a natural relaxant.)

Georgeanne P. Bickle

⌒✐⌒

I have a tip for not waking up in the first place: Get ALL electronic equipment out of the room. It made a huge difference for me.

Donna Cicotte

⌒✐⌒

Slipping off to sleep is a routine I've perfected that's the same every night. I lie down, turn on my left side so I'm facing away from my wife and put a pillow between my legs, with my head between two other pillows, thus making a "head sandwich" to block any extraneous sounds.

I pull the sheets up so they cover half the pillow on top but leave a channel open for my mouth to breathe. After a few moments, I turn flat on my stomach, leaving my right leg splayed out on the pillow at my midsection. I manage to catch the next train to sleepsville in less than five minutes.

Steve Ecclesine

# Why Count Sheep When You Can Sleep?

I have a whole repertoire of dream-like fantasies I use to go to sleep. I'll pick one and play with it until I'm off to sleep. They're completely nonsensical. Some of my favorites:

- I have telekinetic powers and imagine how people would react when I fly things around a room, or I touch someone and know their entire past...and future...or heal children with cancer...or have the ability to pick winning stocks.

- I create all kinds of technology, like solar cold fusion reactors, cyborg military soldiers, satellites. Or I'll discover new planets or develop all kinds of smart new computers.

- I dream about what my life would be like if I won the lottery—what I'd do with all that money and what kind of house I'd live in.

It's all crazy stuff. The crazier it is, the more it resembles your mind when you're sleeping and dreaming. You never want to dwell on real-life issues...they keep me up at night.

Bill Ivie
(Yes, THAT Bill Ivie, the snorer from hell)

POST-BED TIP:

**Keep a sleep diary** for about two weeks to find out what might be causing your sleep problem. A sleep diary should include what time you went to bed, how long it took you to fall asleep and how much coffee you drank during the day. For a complete list of diary items, see www.insomnia123.com by Dr. Mike Steinberg.

## Notes

Techniques that work for you (from the previous list—or new ones you invented):

Other comments:

# Acknowledgements/Resources

I'd like to thank my husband Bill, whose incessant snoring inspired this book, and who remains my deepest friend, despite many sleepless nights. A million thanks to Jim Donovan, best-selling author and book coach, who helped me shape this project from a rough collection of ideas to the book it is today. And to Maria of What's Brewing at Maria's in Frenchtown, New Jersey, for providing such a stimulating atmosphere for hatching ideas.

I'd also like to acknowledge my brothers and sisters, especially Kim and Michele, for their invaluable suggestions, and Bill Miller, who came up with the title. Also thanks to Genevieve LaVo Cosdon, who created such a fabulous cover, and Regina Muster for my photo.

Many thanks to Peter Shankman, founder of Help a Reporter Out (HARO), which put me in contact with so many wonderful people and ideas.

Finally, thank you to everyone who contributed sleep tips. Their ideas were invaluable and I'm deeply indebted. I communicated with some of them so often I almost feel like we're friends. (At the very least, we share a strong personal bond—how many people are willing to confess their intimate secrets to a total stranger?)

Many of the people below are business owners, so I'm

Contributors

including their Web sites, if supplied to me.

Thank you, everyone!

**Contributors:**

Doreen Amatelli
www.waytogoal.com

Peter Archer
www.nmessences.com

Bob Baker
www.nowa.org/profiles/Baker.htm

Susan Barrett

David Berman
www.davidberman.com

Georganne P. Bickle
www.talpub.com

April Biddle

Shannon Cannon

Vince Cardarelli

# Why Count Sheep When You Can Sleep?

Kathi Casey
www.HealthyBoomerBody.com

Donna Cicotte

John Connors

Garen Daly
www.frugalyankee.com

Tom Davis
www.yourremodelingcoach.com

Adrienne Dellwo
chronicfatigue.guide@about.com

Ruthann Disotell
www.celebrationofalifetime.com

Jim Donovan
www.jimdonovan.com

Ed Duffy

Amy Ecclesine

Steve Ecclesine
www.soyouwannabeaproducer.com

# Contributors

Dudley Evenson
www.soundings.com

Ruth Folit
www.lifejournal.com

Jeanna Gabellini
www.masterpeacecoaching.com

Marcella Glenn
http://critiqueandwrite.blogspot.com

Dr. Nancy Irwin
www.drnancyirwin.com

Bill Ivie

Kara L.C. Jones, Dreamer
www.MotherHenna.Etsy.com

Lis King

Renee Kinney
www.millarsalon.com

Amy Logan
PROfusion Publicity

Kathy Loidolt
www.shoppersguidetohealthyliving.com

# Why Count Sheep When You Can Sleep?

James Malone
www.inthenewspr.com

Dr. Sunny Massad
www.hawaiiwellnessinstitute.org

Sharon McPherson
http://twitter.com/SHARONMCP

Natalie McCullough

MaryAnn Miller
www.maryannlmiller.com

Peggy Miller

Jill Nussinow
www.theveggiequeen.com

Jessica Ortner
www.thetappingsolution.com

Sarah Oulman

Wendy Owen
www.insomnia-connection.com

Randy Peyser
www.authoronestop.com

# Contributors

Pine Street Foundation
www.pinestreetfoundation.org

Monica Ricci
www.catalystorganizing.com

Debbie Rittelman
www.dickenslanejewelers.com

Dr. Patricia Ross
www.RobertsRossPublishing.com

Bob Seeley

Scott Shuster
www.scottshuster.com

Jeanne Griffin Smith

Pablo Solomon
www.pablosolomon.com

Maureen Staiano
www.achieveyourdreamcoaching.com

Dr. Mike Steinberg
www.insomnia123.com

Tom Stillman
www.stillmanphoto.com

# Why Count Sheep When You Can Sleep?

Lauren Traub
www.Twifties.com

Terry Traveland
www.ChocolatePrescription.com

Bonnie Vandewater

Charles Wasilewski

Barbara Worton
Author, "BedTime Stories, The short, long and tall tales of a sleepwriter" www.greatlittlebooksllc.com

## About the Author

One of the world's lightest sleepers, Tracy Ecclesine Ivie is a magazine and newspaper editor/writer who learned all about sleeplessness in a noisy Manhattan apartment while being married to the "snorer from hell." She and Bill currently live in central New Jersey and are happily sleeping through the night.

Tracy is also co-author in the book series, "Country Inns of America," and author of the e-book, "How to Get a Merchant Account and Take Credit Card Payments Online and Offline."

www.ingramcontent.com/pod-product-compliance
Lightning Source LLC
Chambersburg PA
CBHW030017290326
41934CB00005B/379